Preventing Cardiovascular Disease in Primary Care
Second Edition

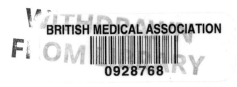

Preventing Cardiovascular Disease in Primary Care

Second Edition

CLIVE HANDLER
BSc, MD, MRCP, FACC, FESC
Consultant in Pulmonary Hypertension
The National Pulmonary Hypertension Service
Royal Free Hospital, London
Consultant Cardiologist
Hospital of St John and St Elizabeth, and Highgate Hospital, London
Honorary Senior Lecturer
Royal Free and University College Medical School, London

and

GERRY COGHLAN
MD, FRCP
Consultant Cardiologist and Director
The National Pulmonary Hypertension Unit, Royal Free Hospital, London

Foreword by
MARIE-ANNE ESSAM
General Practitioner in Hertfordshire, with an interest in Diabetes
Medical Director, South East Essex

Radcliffe Publishing
Oxford • New York

Radcliffe Publishing Ltd
18 Marcham Road
Abingdon
Oxon OX14 1AA
United Kingdom

www.radcliffe-oxford.com
Electronic catalogue and worldwide online ordering facility.

British Library Cataloguing in Publication Data

A catalogue record for this book is available from the British Library.

ISBN-13: 978 184619 145 9

Typeset by Pindar New Zealand (Egan Reid), Auckland, New Zealand
Printed and bound by TJI Digital, Padstow, Cornwall, UK

Contents

Foreword

Here we have colleagues whose lives bear witness to a tireless determination to learn from their patients and to collaborate effectively with colleagues, most especially in primary care.

Drs Handler and Coghlan provide a most readable, rigorous and relevant account of widespread preventable vascular disease, the UK's biggest killer. From pathogenesis, through to pharmacology; from health economics through to patient compliance, this book offers both helicopter and detailed views of its territory.

Comprehensive, case-illustrated explanations of evidence which defines risk, current guidelines and appropriate use of investigations lie within these chapters. Lifestyle and drug treatment of hypertension, dyslipidaemia and obesity are explored. Diabetes and the heart has a chapter all to itself. Stretching from consideration of risk in the young, currently well, through to the complex rehabilitation of comorbid patients, this book is hugely relevant to much of our work in general practice today.

This book takes us further, though, than others on the market. A chapter is devoted to the cutting-edge predictive tool of atheroma imaging. A detailed account is provided of exercise advice best given to people with a variety of cardiac conditions, with accompanying discussion of risks and benefits to the patient. Such information will equip the possessors of this manual with evidence-based counsel for patients, and enable us to engage with them in a reasoned understanding of cardiac rehabilitation.

Whilst acknowledging the crucial role of Government and Public Health in addressing our nation's fate, the crux of success hinges, the authors convince me, on good advice, given well. Drs Handler and Coghlan are listeners. This is evident from exemplary care of deeply appreciative patients, some we shared in common, and from their perceptive account of the causes and consequences of cardiovascular risk. They refer to the 'complex art of giving a patient lifestyle advice which is often not requested and occasionally resented'. This is in the ambiguous context of a consumer-led society where patients want to understand risks and benefits of procedures and treatment.

If any book can help the primary care team get to grips with cardiovascular truth as understood today, if any book can equip us to so connect with our patients we change history with them, this is it.

Dr Marie-Anne Essam
General Practitioner in Hertfordshire, with an interest in Diabetes
Medical Director, South East Essex
May 2008

Preface

Cardiovascular disease is the leading cause of death and disability in the world. Coronary heart disease, an important manifestation of atheromatous vascular disease, accounts for at least 120 000 deaths in the UK each year. Although morbidity and mortality from cardiovascular disease have reduced over the last 25 years (largely due to smoking cessation, treatments for hypertension and dyslipidaemia, and increasing public awareness about diet, obesity and exercise), the incidence of cardiovascular disease and its associated healthcare costs are high in the UK compared to other parts of Europe. Cardiovascular disease is largely preventable and, at the very least, can be delayed by attention to established risk factors. Further reductions in morbidity and mortality are possible, but require public education starting in childhood, incentives for lifestyle modifications, and drug treatments.

There are clear benefits in treating all patients at high risk, particularly those with vascular disease, regardless of the levels of their risk factors. When risk prediction charts are used, younger people usually fall into a low-risk, non-treatment category, even if they have significant risk factors. The optimum management of this large group of patients is unclear. Reducing risk in the population by means of changes in lifestyle and possibly using drugs necessitates collaboration between government and the food and pharmaceutical industries.

Primary care is the natural and most appropriate location for cardiovascular prevention. The tasks for primary care clinicians in this regard are considerable – time-consuming but worthwhile. A large part of their daily work consists of the screening, investigation, treatment and monitoring of patients for both primary and secondary prevention. GPs, practice nurses and other primary healthcare professionals need considerable and continuous support and resources from government for this work.

Patients expect GPs, practice nurses, pharmacists, dieticians and physiotherapists to provide answers about their health concerns. Patients want understandable explanations about why their cholesterol is high and whether they need treatment; how they could improve their diet and how they can lose weight; how much and what type of exercise they can do; how much alcohol they can drink safely and what type of alcohol is advised; whether they really need tablets for their blood pressure and, if they take tablets, whether certain symptoms are due to the tablets. Those who smoke and want to quit want practical and effective help. Diabetics require constant supervision and education. Patients referred for tests and procedures want to know what is involved and what the risks and benefits are.

National and international guidelines for the management of cardiovascular risk factors continue to evolve and are not identical. They serve as a useful basis for treatment but do not and can never replace careful, individualised management for a specific patient sitting in your consulting room. There are new guidelines for treating hypertension with relegation of β-blockers to fourth line, and lower treatment thresholds for hypertension and dyslipidaemia; the indications for angiotensin-converting enzyme inhibitors have expanded. The elderly are grouped together with middle-aged patients and are treated using a similar approach. It is likely that with elucidation of the pathogenesis of atheromatous disease and the identification of high-risk groups, e.g. diabetics, new drugs tackling cardiovascular disease and lower intervention thresholds will emerge.

This book is a companion to our book *Management of Cardiac Problems in Primary Care* (Oxford: Radcliffe Publishing, 2008). We hope that it provides our GP colleagues, other primary care healthcare professionals, medical students, healthcare managers and all those interested and involved in cardiovascular prevention, with an accessible and useful reference and everyday manual.

Clive Handler
Gerry Coghlan
Royal Free Hospital, London
May 2008

About the authors

Dr Clive Handler BSc, MD, MRCP, FACC, FESC is Consultant in Pulmonary Hypertension to The National Pulmonary Hypertension Unit at the Royal Free Hospital, London, and Consultant Cardiologist at The Hospital of St John and St Elizabeth, and Highgate Hospital, London, and Honorary Senior Lecturer in Medicine, Royal Free and University College Medical School. He qualified from Guy's Hospital Medical School and trained in cardiology in London and in Milwaukee, University of Wisconsin, USA. He was previously Consultant Cardiologist at Northwick Park and St Mary's Hospitals, London. He edited *Guy's Hospital – 250 years* in 1975 and his textbook *Cardiology in Primary Care* was published by Radcliffe Publishing in 2004. He is co-editor of *Classic Papers in Coronary Angioplasty* (Springer) with Dr Michael Cleman from Yale University Medical School and co-editor of *Vascular Complications in Human Disease: Mechanisms and Consequences* (Springer), and *Advances in Vascular Medicine* (Springer) with Professor David Abraham, Dr Mick Dashwood and Dr Gerry Coghlan. Together with Dr Gerry Coghlan, he wrote *Management of Cardiac Problems in Primary Care* (Radcliffe Publishing) and *Living with Coronary Disease* (Springer). He has written numerous scientific papers.

Dr Gerry Coghlan MD, FRCP is Consultant Cardiologist and Director of the National Pulmonary Hypertension Unit at the Royal Free Hospital. He trained in Dublin and at Harefield and the Royal Free Hospitals. He is an international authority on pulmonary hypertension and has wide interests in general cardiology, the management of coronary heart disease and coronary angioplasty. He has written several books with Dr Clive Handler as well as scientific papers on pulmonary hypertension and other aspects of cardiology.

Acknowledgements

Clive Handler and Gerry Coghlan would like to acknowledge their colleagues in primary care for collaboration in patient care and for encouraging them to write this second edition.

Clive Handler would like to acknowledge his wife, Caroline, and their three children, Charlotte, Sophie and Julius, for their support during the writing of this book. He would also like to acknowledge the inspiring teaching of Professor Lawrence Cohen MD, Yale University School of Medicine.

Dr Gerry Coghlan would like to acknowledge his wife, Eveleen, and their three sons, Niall, Cathal and Eoin, for their support during the writing of this book.

Developments in cardiovascular disease prevention

ONE

The changing role of primary care in cardiovascular disease

The past decade has seen a seismic shift in the management of cardiovascular conditions. As fund-holding has moved to the primary care sector (managed by Primary Care Trusts), so has responsibility for ensuring equal access to high-quality medical care throughout the patient's care pathway. This places an enormous burden on the primary care team, as it is responsible not only for the care it delivers, but also for ensuring that it purchases quality services for secondary care. In addition, the team must cater for the needs of the whole population, not merely those who come through the door. The primary care physician now lives in a world of targets relating to management of obesity, smoking, cholesterol, blood pressure, heart failure and several other conditions.

The good (bad) old days

The obligations, duties and nature of the work of GPs and primary care nurses have changed considerably over the last 20 years. Home visits and out-of-hours duties have more or less disappeared from the routine work of GPs, except perhaps in isolated rural areas. Whether GPs will again take up these 'traditional' duties is unclear.

Until quite recently, GPs could essentially abandon all responsibility for the management of cardiovascular diseases to the specialist 'expert' if they so wished, for several reasons – both professional and scientific. GPs were not expected to provide specialist services, but were considered to be 'experts' on the 'best way' to treat patients. 'Experts' practised 'eminence-based' rather than evidence-based medicine; they had to because there were no nationally agreed management guidelines.

There were scant long-term epidemiological data to inform GPs about the relevance of individual risk factors. Some of the early large studies produced confusing information. Twenty years ago, there was controversy about the importance of what today are accepted as major risk factors. There was also less incentive to identify patients at high cardiovascular risk, because there were few available treatments. There was little information about the optimal levels of blood pressure, cholesterol and blood sugar. Where treatments were available, for example in type 2 diabetes, there were inadequate data to inform and persuade clinicians about which risk factors were important and should be treated. The same paucity of information applied to management of common cardiac conditions including angina, myocardial infarction and heart failure. The major advances in cardiovascular disease prevention and management, which younger clinicians take for granted, have occurred in the last 25 years.

Service provision

Rationing of healthcare could simply be managed through waiting lists. As there was no agreement on how to administer optimal cardiac care, the quality of and waiting times for services varied widely between hospitals just a few miles apart, depending on local 'expert' advice and management competence. Lapses in care were considered to be the responsibility of secondary care. There was, therefore, little incentive for or expectation of GPs to try to improve the situation, and there were no levers available to those who recognised the limitations of care delivery.

Drivers for change: guidelines and audit

In the 1970s, politicians and the public became increasingly disgruntled about the fact that there appeared to be no mechanisms for ensuring that recognised standards of care could be delivered. Similar levels of funding appeared to produce very disparate levels of care in different areas of the country. By the mid-1990s it was absolutely clear that the NHS was failing to deliver first-world-quality healthcare. However, despite the shortcomings of the new system, compared with the situation 10 years ago, high-quality care is now available to a much larger proportion of the population.

Throughout the 1980s and 1990s, large, randomised, controlled studies provided convincing evidence of the value of drug and other treatments in a variety of conditions. This led to a proliferation of guidelines on disease management. These allow clinicians and healthcare managers to evaluate whether treatments are justified and cost-effective, and whether service delivery is 'up to standard'. Questions including: Does the patient need to be referred to a specialist? Does the patient need to be treated in a hospital by a specialist? What investigations should be performed? What is the most appropriate and cost-effective treatment? are now addressed in several national and international practice guidelines. Guidelines have become an integral part of all areas of clinical practice and the management mindset of clinicians in Europe and the USA.

Clinical audit was introduced a few years ago to allow healthcare professionals to measure and demonstrate their performance against agreed standards, introduce measures to improve their performance and re-check their performance in order to 'close the audit loop'. Audit is a difficult discipline but it helps clinicians think about how they can improve their clinical practice and service, and provides objective information to help justify changes.

The NSF and all that

The National Service Framework (NSF) documents changed our world dramatically. Here, for the first time, we had the Government and medical experts agreeing on measurable standards of care that should be delivered. This contracted the Government to paying for a certain level of care, and the medical community to ensuring that this level of care would be delivered. Of course, the Government is committed to achieving this at the least possible cost, so there was a drive, largely based on cost, to deliver as much care as possible in primary care. This has been facilitated by the development of usually robust, evidence-based clinical management guidelines and new service delivery; for example, chest-pain clinics and nurse-delivered domiciliary care for heart failure.

Preventative care in the community based on global risk estimation

The aims of prevention are to reduce the risk of heart attack or stroke, to reduce the need for revascularisation in all arterial territories, and to improve the quality and length of life. Chapter 2 of the NSF requires all primary care practices to assess the cardiovascular risk profile of their patients. Non-pharmacological or 'lifestyle' advice is recommended for all. Drugs to reduce thrombosis, blood pressure, lipids and glucose are used if non-pharmacological methods are inadequate.

Practices should audit the outcome of smoking cessation, and achieve targets for blood pressure and lipids. Weight loss is easy to measure; diet and exercise are less easy to measure, but important in prevention.

Global risk of cardiovascular disease

It is recommended that all adults aged over 40 years who are not already on treatment, and who have no history of cardiovascular disease or diabetes, should have global risk estimation. In addition, global cardiovascular risk should be estimated in people with a family history of premature cardiovascular disease, or with symptoms suggestive of cardiovascular disease. This should include ethnicity, smoking history, family history of cardiovascular disease, weight and waist measurements, blood pressure, non-fasting lipids, and non-fasting glucose. In the UK, people's 10-year cardiovascular risk is estimated using the Joint British Societies' risk charts. In Europe, SCORE tables are used. These provide an approximate estimated probability based on five risk factors: age, gender, smoking, systolic blood pressure, and the ratio of total cholesterol : HDL cholesterol (total cholesterol in mainland Europe).

People with established cardiovascular disease or diabetes, those with high levels of one or more risk factors, and apparently healthy individuals who are at high risk (>20% risk over 10 years) of developing atherosclerotic disease, should be treated equally. All their risk factors should be treated. Initially, patients with a 10-year risk of more than 30% were to receive treatment; this has been reduced to include those with a 10-year risk of more than 20%.

The concept of global or total cardiovascular risk is sensible and practical. It has always, even subconsciously, underpinned clinical management decisions. In the same way as clinicians look at the 'whole patient' before recommending medical or surgical treatments when balancing the risk and the benefit of any intervention – whether aspirin or an aortic valve replacement – global risk estimation helps clinicians and patients make balanced decisions about preventative strategies and treatments. Total risk, based on all risk factors, rather than a single risk factor, is assessed. This is because cardiovascular disease is multifactorial; the presence of more than one risk factor is multiplicative and not additive, and risk factors tend to be associated or are clustered. Even if a target for one risk factor cannot be reached, a patient's global risk can still be reduced by treating other risk factors. Nevertheless, treatment of a high single risk factor is necessary.

Lifestyle advice for all

All people should have lifestyle advice, irrespective of their global risk. Low-risk individuals should be reassessed annually depending on their age. Those at high risk should have lifestyle advice and treatment of individual risk factors.

Lipids

Statins have revolutionised the management of hypercholesterolaemia and have made a considerable difference to the prognosis of patients with vascular disease, and the clinical outcomes in all age groups.

Patients with a total cholesterol : HDL cholesterol ratio of >6.0 mmol/l should be treated with lifestyle and dietary advice, and a statin. People with familial hyperlipidaemia should be treated with a statin. An LDL-cholesterol target of <2.5 mmol/l (<2.0 mmol/l in the USA, and some parts of Europe) for those with vascular disease and 3 mmol/l for primary prevention have provided simple, auditable targets.

Hypertension

Stepped therapy for hypertension (calcium channel blockers, ACE inhibitors and diuretics), has provided a logical sequence of drugs to be prescribed before patients are referred to secondary care.

Simple guidelines for therapy (all patients with a persistent level above 160/100 mmHg and those above 140/90 mmHg who have end-organ damage, or a greater than 20% 10-year risk), identify the population to treat.

Treatment targets (<140/85 mmHg for most patients, and <130/80 mmHg for diabetics) have simplified and standardised management. Lower treatment targets in high-risk patients reinforce the concept of global risk and more aggressive intervention to achieve more stringent targets in high-risk patients.

Service organisation and delivery of care

Service delivery for cardiovascular prevention has required major reorganisation of primary care services. As most of this care is protocol-driven, nurse-led clinics have been set up throughout the country. Computerisation of practices and live database entry has made it possible to simplify audit. Regular audit meetings are held by most practices to ensure that standards are being met. Limited resources have forced clinicians and healthcare managers to question the merits and necessity of traditional practices, which sometimes make life uncomfortable and uneasy for patients, doctors and nurses.

Primary care clinics are now established in railway stations in the UK to offer ease of access to medical advice to people who work and have difficulty finding time to see their GP during working hours. Continuity of care and availability of patients' medical records are problems encountered by such clinics, but are not insurmountable.

In-store primary care clinics are becoming more common in the USA. They are less expensive with low overheads because staffing and estate costs are low and are shared by the store. Appointments are almost immediate with a walk-in service offered, and this is more convenient for patients. But physicians express concern about quality of care. This type of clinic is staffed by nurse practitioners and provide only certain services (for example, vaccination; infections treatment; lipid screening; pregnancy tests; wart removal; bladder, chest, ear and throat infection treatment; minor sunburn treatment) which they feel do not require physician evaluation. The menu items are diagnoses and this puts more of the onus on patients to take responsibility for their health. Patients with important conditions are referred immediately to hospital emergency departments, but this assumes that these conditions are correctly diagnosed. Nurse-led, protocol-based triage is established in accident and emergency departments and so this potential problem is manageable.

NHS Direct and nurse-run, protocol-based decision-making services in UK primary care offer a similar concept of service. A similar model of in-store clinics could work in the UK.

GPs with a special interest in cardiology

The Department of Health advocates the use of GPs with a special interest (GPSI) in cardiology to improve access to cardiology services in the community. A national training and accreditation programme is being developed. The scheme has been endorsed by the British Cardiovascular Society, the Royal College of General Practitioners, the Royal College of Physicians, the Royal College of Nursing, the Primary Care Cardiovascular Society and the British Society of Echocardiography. It is not yet known whether this service will be popular with GPs or what the cost-effectiveness and clinical outcomes will be.

Specialist advice for dyslipidaemia, hypertension and diabetes

Secondary care is now recommended only for those with complex lipid abnormalities (familial hyperlipidaemia, some endocrine associated dyslipidaemia) and for the more complex hypertensive patients (unsatisfactory control despite three or more different medications; secondary hypertension – for example, hypertension during pregnancy; and young patients – below the age of 25 years).

The NSF for diabetes has also cleared the way for most diabetics to be managed in the community, setting simple strategies for regular assessment of complications and simple goals for therapy (HbA$_1$c <6.5%). Specialist referral is now necessary only for the minority of patients with type 2 diabetes.

> Diabetes is a powerful risk factor for cardiovascular disease. There are lower prevention treatment thresholds for diabetic patients.

Chronic care in the community

Recognition that secondary care centres delivered inadequate, unsatisfactory and inefficient care for chronic conditions has led to primary care clinicians taking on this increasingly important role. Conditions like coronary heart disease and heart failure are punctuated by acute episodes that necessitate hospital admission or augmented care. However, for most patients living with these conditions, hospital visits are an inconvenience; only those requiring specialist evaluation, complex investigations or a fundamental change to their treatment need to be referred to hospital.

> Cardiovascular prevention is a fundamental part of the management of cardiac conditions.

Angina and acute coronary syndromes

The precise diagnosis of these conditions remains essentially the preserve of secondary care. Rapid-access chest-pain clinic assessments exclude angina in most patients in a single hospital visit. Those with probable angina can be stratified into low and high risk based on their clinical profile and exercise test results, and arrangements for intervention planned. Once a patient has a firm diagnosis, and any necessary intervention has been undertaken, one moves to a more chronic phase of disease management, where optimisation of risk factors and simple therapies (aspirin, β-blockers, nitrates, calcium channel blockers, and/or nicorandil) are all that are required. Secondary care facilities are then required only for acute episodes (unstable angina and myocardial infarction), and for the relatively small group of patients in whom conventional therapies fail to deliver an adequate quality of life because of poorly controlled angina.

Heart failure

The availability of a blood test for heart failure (BNP or NT-proBNP), which can be requested in primary care, has revolutionised the assessment of breathless patients. However, heart failure clinics remain an essential part of secondary care services. Echocardiography is currently performed mainly in secondary care but should be widely available in primary care. Establishing whether a patient has heart failure and if so, identifying the cause – poor pump function (systolic failure), impaired pump relaxation (diastolic failure) or another underlying heart problem, for example, valvar heart disease – has implications for immediate and long-term management. These problems can be managed, with remote secondary care input or outreach services, in primary care.

The expanding role of internal cardioverter defibrillators (ICDs) for the prevention of sudden death, and biventricular pacing for advanced heart failure (cardiac resynchroni-sation therapy), as well as the recognition of familial forms of dilated cardiomyopathy, and the role of revascularisation for some patients with ischaemic heart failure, means that precise diagnosis is important for most patients once heart failure has been established as a diagnosis. However, as in the case of angina, for the majority of patients, once secondary care has finished playing with their 'toys', chronic care is best delivered in the community. Ensuring that patients with heart failure are on ACE inhibitors and β-blockers has become an important target for primary care clinicians.

The community heart failure nurse has a pivotal role in ensuring that spironolactone is used safely in patients with advanced heart failure, performing and checking blood test results for possible haematological and biochemical abnormalities, ensuring that low-sodium diets are adhered to, and advising patients to weigh themselves daily, exercise regularly, and modify their diuretic dosage according to weight changes (and supervising that they do so).

Atrial fibrillation

Most arrhythmias have become firmly the province of secondary care, but not atrial fibrillation. Atrial flutter and supraventricular tachycardia can be cured by ablation; bradyarrhythmias are treated with pacing; implantable cardioverter defibrillators are used to treat serious ventricular arrhythmias. Years ago cardioversion was widely practised for the management of atrial fibrillation, but it has been recognised that such efforts are in vain, as rate control and anticoagulation give the same quality of life and prognosis for the majority of patients.

Patients should be investigated and treated for underlying causes, particularly hypertension.

In those requiring a more aggressive approach, radio-frequency ablation is generally a better option. Ablation for atrial fibrillation is, however, a tedious and frequently unsuccessful undertaking and, as the left atrium must be entered, these procedures are associated with a modest risk of stroke. Therefore, ablation of atrial fibrillation remains a procedure for patients whose symptoms are not satisfactorily controlled with one, or a combination, of digoxin, verapramil, β-blockers, and amiodarone.

The role of anticoagulation for atrial fibrillation probably does necessitate some secondary care involvement. While many GP surgeries can monitor warfarin, the decision to start long-term warfarin to reduce the risk of thromboembolic complications has to be individualised, but patients should have a risk-factor assessment. In essence, low-risk patients (<1% per annum stroke risk: age <65, with a normal-sized and normally functioning heart on echocardiography, and who have no thyroid dysfunction, who are normotensive, and have no history of embolic phenomena) should not be anticoagulated. High-risk patients (>5% per annum risk: those with embolic phenomena especially within the previous 12 months; those with poor left ventricular systolic function; those with significant valvular lesions, especially mitral stenosis), should be anticoagulated unless there are significant risks of bleeding, or major logistical problems with monitoring. But the majority of patients fit into the intermediate group, where rules become fuzzy, such as: age over 70 years, a normal left ventricle, and no significant valve lesion. However, once the decision has been made, secondary care has little to add to the management of these patients, and patients can be appropriately monitored in primary care and referred back for a specialist review when necessary.

Murmurs and valvular heart disease

Hospital consultants have a long history of collecting 'valve' patients for the purposes of teaching medical students, and as examination fodder. This has been justified on the basis that such conditions may deteriorate asymptomatically to a point beyond which surgery is safe. This is clearly true for regurgitant lesions, and there is a growing body of evidence to support the belief that aortic stenosis, too, may cause symptoms that are not noted by the patient, but are elucidated during exercise testing. Therefore, in the setting of significant valve disease, the involvement of secondary care is justified unless a primary care group has a general practitioner with special interest (GPSI) who has been specifically trained in managing valvular heart disease patients, and is competent to manage these patients.

Generally, patients with heart murmurs are increasingly the preserve of primary care. In most cases, an 'open-access' echocardiogram to demonstrate either that there is no valve lesion, or that the degree of abnormality is minor, will reassure the patient and the referring GP that the patient does not need to be either referred or followed up in hospital. However, some patients should be carefully flagged and followed up in primary care and referred for serial echocardiography depending on their symptoms. Patients with aortic stenosis may need follow-up depending on their valve area and aortic valve gradient. Similarly, patients with important mitral stenosis and/or mitral regurgitation, and aortic regurgitation should be followed up jointly by both the GP and a cardiologist.

> Treating cardiovascular risk factors is an important part of the management of aortic valve stenosis.

Open-access echocardiography is available to most primary care physicians. So long as reporting is sufficiently detailed and includes management advice and guidelines for referral, secondary care need not be involved in a large proportion of patients with valvular heart disease. An adequate report should comment on any valvular abnormalities detected – whether these are within the range of normality (for example, 70% of people have mild tricuspid regurgitation) or abnormal; if abnormal, does this abnormality require antibiotic prophylaxis during future potentially septic procedures, and what, if any, follow-up is necessary (for example, a repeat echo in five years' time for a patient with aortic sclerosis).

Rare conditions and tertiary care

Rare conditions like hypertrophic cardiomyopathy, Marfan's syndrome, most congenital cardiac lesions, familial risk of sudden cardiac death, and pulmonary arterial hypertension should always be the preserve of tertiary care.

The brave new world

The clarification of the roles of primary versus secondary and tertiary care in the management of cardiovascular disease should lead to much higher-quality service. Care that needs to be delivered to the entire population (risk assessment and management) can be delivered only by primary care. Chronic disease management for common conditions (for example, 10% of the older population have atrial fibrillation, coronary heart disease, and heart failure) is best delivered close to the patient's home. In turn, secondary care must concentrate on delivering efficiently those aspects of care that require a high level of expertise (echocardiography, angioplasty, cardiac surgery and electrophysiology), or treating conditions which require management not easily delivered by prescribed protocol-driven care.

An obvious consequence of the paradigm shift from medicine as an art form (with unquantifiable benefits) to a business model (delivering 'x' amount of care to 'y' people in 'z' time frame) is that we can now plan care delivery, and explore and refine models of care. This has already led to a substantial expansion of nurse-led clinics both in primary care and in hospitals, and has changed the nature of the doctor-patient relationship forever.

As one works through the care delivery package and the working relationships between the various professionals involved, it will become apparent that although the model starts off with clear lines of responsibility, the role of professional judgement has not diminished – it has merely moved to more defined decision points. The patient now has expectations in terms of waiting times, being treated courteously, and standards of care, but still relies on our judgement and humanity.

FURTHER READING

Bohmer R. The Rise of In-Store Clinics – Threat or Opportunity? *N Engl J Med.* 2007; **356:** 765–8.

Organisation of prevention services in primary care

TWO

Economic implications of cardiovascular disease in the UK

Cardiovascular disease is the major cause of death in developed countries. It caused 40% of all deaths (238,000) in the UK in 2002; 50% of these were due to coronary heart disease and 30% due to cerebrovascular disease. Death often results suddenly and prematurely, before medical care and interventions are available. Angina, myocardial infarction and acute coronary syndromes often result when the disease is advanced and when the costs and risks of treatment are high.

> Cardiovascular disease is strongly related to lifestyle. Most of the risk factors are modifiable. Risk-factor modification, particularly in high-risk individuals, reduces morbidity and mortality.

Cardiovascular disease-related healthcare costs, including community and social services, accident and emergency care, hospital care, rehabilitation and drugs, and non-healthcare costs due to productivity losses, have been estimated to have cost the UK economy £29 billion in 2004. Sixty per cent of the total costs of cardiovascular disease (£17.4 billion) are consumed by healthcare. This proportion is the highest of any country in the European Union, including Germany and France. Twenty-three per cent of the costs were due to loss of productivity due to mortality and morbidity.

Epidemiology of coronary heart disease in the UK

The incidence of coronary heart disease in the UK is among the highest in the world. The mortality rate from coronary heart disease is higher in Scotland than in the south of England, and higher in people of lower socio-economic class. It is not clear whether this is a causal effect or due to lifestyle habits – an unhealthy diet causing obesity with associated hypertension, diabetes and dyslipidaemia, smoking and lack of effective cardiovascular exercise.

> Atherosclerosis develops insidiously over many years and is often advanced before symptoms occur.
>   Risk-factor modifications have been shown to reduce cardiovascular mortality and morbidity, particularly in high-risk subjects.

The prevalence of coronary heart disease is higher in people from Southern Asia. The cause of this is unclear but has been suggested to be due to insulin resistance and a higher prevalence of the metabolic syndrome.

The changing role and greater responsibility of primary care in cardiovascular disease prevention

Primary and secondary prevention of cardiovascular disease constitute a large part of the work in primary care. More patients with cardiovascular disease are being diagnosed, investigated, treated and followed up in primary care, for a number of reasons. These include National Health Service policies and targets for primary care, and a logistical and cost-based decision for placing greater responsibility for cardiovascular prevention on primary care physicians and nurses. The role of primary care in cardiovascular prevention, as well as in other cardiac conditions, will probably increase as a fewer patients are followed up in hospital clinics.

In addition to encouraging patients and their families to stop smoking; to eat a healthier, low-fat, low-salt diet; to lose weight, and to take frequent, regular, useful exercise, primary care clinicians have a responsibility to screen for, and where necessary, intervene in patients with these risk factors. This is time consuming.

The availability of cholesterol testing in pharmacies and cheaper statins 'over the counter' may encourage wider use of these drugs in people who currently do not fulfil criteria for treatment paid for by the NHS. This will probably increase the work in primary care because patients will need clinical advice and biochemical monitoring.

There has also been a lowering of the treatment threshold and a change in the recommendations for monitoring and treating hypertension. Obesity is an increasing problem in the Western world and particularly in the UK. This, too, will occupy time and is another challenge for primary care. Smoking cessation and obesity clinics also offer opportunities to primary care clinicians to reduce cardiovascular risk in their communities.

> Cardiovascular disease is strongly related to lifestyle and modifiable factors. Assessing and treating all individual risk factors reduces total cardiovascular risk.

Primary care clinicians also have a broader responsibility for providing advice in other areas of lifestyle and health. This is worthwhile and professionally satisfying work. Utilising the talents and enthusiasm of patient groups, chefs, dieticians, pharmacists, physiotherapists and exercise trainers, spreads a culture and atmosphere of health promotion in the community and reinforces and supplements medical advice.

Effective cardiovascular prevention works best with a well-organised, multidisciplinary system for screening and identifying patients who are likely to benefit from repeated education about lifestyle and pharmacological interventions. Most adults understand the concept of cardiovascular risk factors. However, effective prevention depends on people taking responsibility for their health and putting these messages into practice.

Conventional risk factors for atherosclerosis account for the vast majority of cardio-vascular disease and most people accept this. Making long-term changes in lifestyle is difficult irrespective of socio-economic or educational class, particularly for people with no known vascular disease. This is because, generally, they do not have symptoms and because the relationship between risk factors and individual risk is neither completely consistent nor immediate. The presence or absence of risk factors in individuals does not precisely predict outcomes because the impact of risk factors in different individuals is variable and dependent on indeterminate factors such as duration of exposure and differing susceptibility. Even people who have coronary heart disease and who have had a heart attack find it difficult to continue the lifestyle changes they started with determination and vigour in the cardiac care unit.

Approach to cardiovascular prevention in primary care

Primary care clinicians have a major role in educating patients and their families. In order for patients to be interested, active, responsible, and dedicated participants in reducing their cardiovascular risk they must understand:
✧ why prevention is important
✧ that a healthy lifestyle is for life
✧ what cardiovascular risk factors are
✧ which risk factors they can modify
✧ the likely consequences and implications if they do not adhere to a healthy lifestyle
✧ what they have to do to reduce their risk
✧ how the primary care team can help and support them.

Primary care clinicians have to understand the patient's:
✧ perspective of their health and what they want for their future
✧ ability and willingness to help themselves
✧ social and personal circumstances which impinge on their ability to follow a healthy lifestyle.

Factors which make it difficult for patients to change their lifestyle

✧ Depression, anxiety, low self-esteem.
✧ Entrenched beliefs.
✧ Loneliness, social isolation.
✧ Uncontrolled lifestyle, irregular hours at work.
✧ Stress.

Educating the young to take responsibility for their health

Childhood obesity increases the risk of cardiovascular disease in adulthood.
Cardiovascular prevention is more likely to be successful if children are taught about healthy lifestyles. Children have sexual health education lessons in school. These should be expanded to include cardiovascular health. Children should be taught the practicalities of

cardiovascular health prevention, and this could include food shopping choices and food preparation. Children should be encouraged to teach their parents about cardiovascular prevention. Primary care clinicians rather than school teachers may be the most effective people to teach school children about health issues.

Healthy habits should be encouraged and made easy and affordable so that they can be continued. This necessitates co-operation and collaboration between government and industry. This principle also applies to explaining the risks of smoking, alcohol, and illegal drugs.

Diabetes, obesity, a high-fat diet, an inactive lifestyle, and hypertension (which is often associated with these conditions) are becoming more common in Britain. Smoking is probably becoming less common among adults, particularly in socio-economic class I. It is likely that the smoking ban in public places in the UK will result in further reductions in the number of people smoking.

> A major part of the work of primary care clinicians is cardiovascular disease prevention. This time-consuming work demands efficient organisation and enthusiasm.
>
> Patient education, encouragement and continued monitoring of risk factors are required to reduce cardiovascular risk.

Clinicians caring for patients with cardiovascular disease can appreciate the beneficial secondary preventive effects of cardio-preventive drugs on individual patients. The direct primary preventive effects of these drugs are less easy to assess in large populations. Age-adjusted mortality rates for cardiovascular disease have decreased but this may not be due solely to drugs for cardiovascular prevention.

Primary care collaborative services and patient self-help groups

The majority of GP surgeries and larger primary care clinics currently run independently from other practices and the local hospital. In some parts of Britain, it may be convenient and cost effective for primary care clinicians from different practices to provide collaborative prevention clinics. A GP and/or practice nurse, together with staff interested in obesity and diet, exercise, and smoking, could join forces, possibly with suitable lay people who may be patients of the practice, to provide ongoing leadership and support to patient self-help groups. After training, the patients could run their own meetings – endorsed, supported and supervised by the primary care clinicians. This system could cascade to other patient groups and practices. This type of clinic allows patients to share experiences and learn from one another. Patient groups provide support and encouragement, energise the staff and strengthen the practice.

People of all ages (particularly the young) in the community, should be educated about cardiovascular disease, the risk factors, the consequences, and how they may reduce their chances of developing coronary heart disease and stroke. This is particularly relevant for secondary prevention, where patients can share their experiences and support other patients who have had heart attacks and myocardial revascularisation.

Primary care cardiovascular physicians

A logical consequence of the increasingly prominent role of primary care physicians in managing patients with cardiovascular problems is the growing number of GPs with a cardiovascular interest (GP with a special interest – GPSI). They have established themselves as a large, active and academic group. The Primary Care Cardiovascular Society is an active and valued affiliated group of the British Cardiac Society. Diploma courses, conferences, further education with GPs working with specialists in hospital clinics, will produce a large number of interested GPs with enhanced training and experience in cardiology, able to provide an increasingly skilled and broad specialist service for their patients.

Polyclinics

In the days of fundholding, some GPs established cardiology outreach clinics where a consultant cardiologist worked with the GP in the surgery to provide a joint consultation service. This had several advantages. Patients preferred to see the specialist in their GP surgery rather than attend a hospital where it is uncommon for patients to see the same doctor on each visit. Databases containing patient records linked between primary care and the hospital investigation services are important parts of the infrastructure. Local community polyclinics are the logical successor of outreach clinics and have the following potential benefits:

⬥ The GP can discuss the patient face-to-face with the cardiologist. GP referral letters to specialists become redundant and therefore cannot be lost in the hospital postal and filing system.
⬥ Patients are more likely to attend the appointment because attending the GP surgery is easier, quicker, cheaper, more personal and less intimidating than attending hospital. There should be a lower non-attendance rate.
⬥ There may be fewer inappropriate referrals for open-access investigations with consequent cost savings and more efficient use of resources. The total number of investigations requests, however, may be greater.
⬥ Combined primary care and specialist clinics provide a two-way learning experience and help forge helpful professional relationships based on an understanding of the primary care–secondary care interface and a collegiate relationship.
⬥ Joint community clinics bring doctors together and provide an opportunity for research and audit, development of protocols for investigation and treatment, and a forum for informed and sensible discussion of how healthcare delivery can be developed and refined in the future.
⬥ Most non-invasive cardiac investigations can be done in the polyclinic.

The resource implications are unclear.

The changing face of patients

Primary care is undergoing a revolution. Patients are more interested and knowledgeable and have higher expectations of doctors, nurses and the health service.

Patients may have significant misunderstandings and inappropriate fears about their cardiovascular health. Patients consult the internet and read medical books. Their most likely source of medical advice (other than a doctor or a nurse) is a friend willing to share their own, often unrelated problems and experiences. This lay advice is often the source of misunderstanding and confusion, but it is unavoidable.

Primary care clinicians should feel comfortable to discuss all aspects of a patient's condition. Sex, diet and exercise are common sources of anxiety which patients may be embarrassed to discuss.

Patients are increasingly likely to have a consultation with a nurse rather than a doctor. They may want the answers to specific lifestyle questions as well as advice about their symptoms. Patients are more informed, more likely to question the advice given and less prepared to wait to see a specialist or have an investigation.

Many GPs are now expert in primary and secondary prevention of coronary heart disease and are being encouraged to develop their interests and skills in cardiology. Some are providing specialist services in hospital cardiac departments. Nurses are also playing an increasingly important diagnostic and therapeutic role in both primary care and hospital.

Non-medical prescribing

Since May 2006, certain nurses and pharmacist prescribers are allowed to prescribe any licensed medicine (except most controlled drugs) within their sphere of competence.

Communication: understanding the patient and getting the prevention message across clearly and simply

Communication is the key component of medical practice. This is of particular importance in cardiovascular prevention.

Understanding and listening to the patient

It is difficult to give any clinical advice without a good understanding of the patient's history and relevant medical history, all their risk factors, their family history, their drug/medication history and their level of activity, and physical findings. This is as important in cardiovascular prevention as in other disciplines.

It is important to understand the patient's perspective of their health, their personal views on whether they are willing and able to make necessary and often difficult changes to the way they live their lives.

Is the patient prepared to change to a healthy lifestyle?

Clinicians generally believe that most patients want to live longer and are interested in eating a healthy diet, learning about the benefits of exercise and possibly doing some exercise, and learning what things they can do for themselves to lower their risk of heart disease. Some patients, however, are not interested in prevention. They may not be willing or able to change their lifestyle and compromise their enjoyment of life for the potential gain of a longer, healthier, more productive and enjoyable future. The view of 'live for the day' is widespread in young people who, although may be at low risk, are an important group who benefit from cardiovascular prevention.

Despite television and radio programmes, articles in the press and popular magazines, and advice from primary care clinicians, a large proportion of patients cannot connect with the idea, and certainly not the practice, of cardiovascular disease prevention. This frame of mind is perhaps most common in children and young adults, who do not think about their mortality and feel immune from cardiovascular disease. Older patients often think that it is too late or not possible to change their lifestyle at their time of life, even though they are at highest risk and have the most to gain from risk reduction.

Giving prevention advice to patients who do not understand or who are not interested may be considered a waste of time. It is therefore important to understand the patient's viewpoint before embarking on prevention management.

Understanding each other

Where patients speak a different language from the clinician, it is essential to get an interpreter (who may be a family member). This can be difficult in primary care. Practices based in areas where communication is a problem may need to seek the help of their Primary Care Trust for advice, or members of the community who may be able to provide interpreters.

Explaining the principles of prevention

It is important that patients understand the reasons and the potential benefits of making major changes to their lifestyle. Although most people now accept that smoking is dangerous, that high blood pressure increases the risk of stroke and heart attacks, and that diabetes increases the risks of arterial problems, reiteration of these messages is more likely to result in effective lifestyle changes than a single, hurried discussion. This information should be conveyed enthusiastically and with conviction but patients should not be pressurised or browbeaten; this can be counterproductive. Patients should be given factual information clearly and positively so that they can then make up their own mind on how they wish to proceed.

Risk-factor clinics

Most GPs run clinics for smoking cessation, high blood pressure, obesity, lipids, and diabetes, but few run dedicated exercise clinics. This important part of prevention is usually mentioned as part of the package of prevention measures and is certainly a key part of cardiac rehabilitation.

Effective risk-factor clinics depend on patients' understanding of the principles of prevention. They should understand the impact that they can make on their future. This usually takes more than a one-off consultation. Patients are more likely to make long-term modifications to the way they live their lives after an enthusiastic, persuasive and empathic consultation, with messages expressed simply and clearly.

> It takes a lot of time, enthusiasm and commitment to run worthwhile prevention clinics.

Are tablets necessary?

Most people would rather take a tablet to help them stop smoking or lose weight than go through the agonies of self-discipline. Tablets to aid smoking cessation are of limited efficacy. Diet tablets are rarely used. Older formulations were withdrawn as they caused pulmonary hypertension. A low-fat diet is cheaper than statins but comparatively ineffective in lowering cholesterol.

Tablets have side effects. They have a cost. Tablets should be offered to patients who would benefit significantly. Evidence-based prescribing is helpful and reassuring but not possible in all patients. In these cases, treatment has to be prescribed on an individual basis.

Long-term support and encouragement

In obese patients, weight loss and exercise may be sufficient without the need for tablets, to lower mild hypertension. Although it is easier and quicker for doctors to prescribe medication, providing education and encouragement to patients to change their diet and lose weight, stop smoking, and take regular exercise, is preferable. It is cheaper and there is no associated risk of drug-induced side effects.

Patients who can successfully modify their risk factors without tablets are more likely to achieve long-term benefits than those who cannot. Most patients will require long-term support and encouragement because of the high risk of regressing back to old habits. This is particularly the case with exercise which, when done properly to achieve cardiovascular fitness, may not be enjoyable – 'no pain, no gain'. However, regular, daily exercise is an important and effective measure in cardiovascular disease prevention. It has many benefits but demands considerable discipline and commitment.

The patient's perspective: what do patients want from their GP?

Patients want the opportunity and time to explain how they feel and what they are worried about. They want their doctor to listen, understand, and take them and their concerns seriously. They want reassurance, help, advice and a sympathetic explanation of their symptoms. Although it is not usually possible for patients to have lengthy consultations, patients can usually discuss their problems with their GP or the practice nurse on another visit.

If investigations or specialist consultations are necessary, patients do not want to wait a long time for them. Most patients are aware that delays may be outside the control of the GP. However, their anxiety may override their sympathy for the GP who is expected to deliver prompt, high-quality medical services in the face of prolonged waiting times, ever-changing organisational issues and 'targets', and resource restrictions imposed on both the primary care team and the hospital service. Patients want all aspects of their medical care to be carried out quickly. They may want to see a specialist even when the GP may not think this necessary. Patients want to feel better quickly.

What does the primary healthcare team need to do?

The primary healthcare team has a difficult generalist and specialist role including diagnosis, referring patients to the appropriate specialist, and explaining test results and specialist management plans to patients and, sometimes, justifying these to healthcare managers. GPs are expected to prescribe drugs in accordance with local therapeutic committee guidelines.

Primary care clinicians have to listen to the patient, understand what the patient needs and try to help them. Patients must be treated courteously, with respect and made to feel at ease and allowed to ask the clinician questions. These should be answered openly, honestly and sensitively. This is difficult in the restricted time available in most busy GP practices.

Talking to worried patients whose fear, desperation or confusion may occasionally transpose to anger is an art. The primary healthcare team needs to have the resources, time, energy, training and ability to cope with patients' demands and increasing expectations. All those involved in the care of patients with cardiovascular problems should have the necessary knowledge and skills.

Some patients have a 'hidden agenda' or secret fears about their health prompted by the illness of a friend or member of the family and it is important to elicit this. Their symptoms may be a manifestation of anxiety related to their personal or family life, or business situation and the GP and nurse are usually in an advantageous position to analyse the problem. This may be all that is required to help the patient.

The nurse practitioner

Nurse practitioners are increasingly important members of the primary healthcare team and play a prominent part in patient care, performing many parts of the traditional doctor's role. Patients generally like the idea of seeing a nurse in primary care and trust their professional ability.

Cardiovascular risk assessment and treatment, weight reduction, diet and dietary supplements and personal lifestyle advice, including advice on smoking, alcohol use, exercise and sex are important and common aspects of cardiology in primary care. Nurses, therefore, need to have a sound knowledge of the role of these factors in clinical care. They may also be engaged in clinical evaluation and so will need to be able to take a cardiac history, examine the patient, and make a diagnosis in collaboration with the GP. Together, with an understanding of cardiac tests, they should feel confident in drawing up a management plan and knowing which patients should be referred for specialist opinion.

Other members of the primary healthcare team

Pharmacists, dieticians, physiotherapists and complementary medical specialists play an increasingly prominent role in primary care and each have an integrated role in different conditions.

Pharmacists

Patients often ask their pharmacists about tablets and symptoms which they think could be drug side effects. This is a difficult issue. If in any doubt, pharmacists should advise patients to discuss the problem with the GP who prescribed the medication. Patients are often concerned and confused about possible side effects from drugs used for cardiovascular prevention.

Pharmacists make it easier for patients to take tablets. They provide pill dispensers, deliver medication to patients' homes, explain why they should be taking the tablets, and check compliance. Dose adjustments in the elderly and those with renal or liver impairment, and simplification of treatment and dosage regimes to improve compliance, are key areas where pharmacists make major improvements to clinical care and lighten the workload for the GP.

Dieticians

Dieticians have expertise to help patients lose weight, improve diabetic control, hypertension and hyperlipidaemia. Patients may want to know whether new dietary supplements and vitamins are beneficial and what food is beneficial or harmful. Vitamin supplements are not necessary for people who eat a balanced diet. Alcohol is popular and patients may be confused about its value and dangers in their particular condition and how much and what type they should drink.

Physiotherapists

Physiotherapists have specialised knowledge and skills in a range of conditions. Their advice and encouragement to patients to exercise regularly are important. Exercise is of proven benefit to patients for both primary and secondary prevention and for patients with heart failure. Exercise and rehabilitation should be available in primary care.

Dental care

Patients with structural heart defects and heart valve conditions should have good oral hygiene and have access to a dentist knowledgeable about the evolving indications for antibiotic prophylaxis and dental assessments before valve surgery.

Complementary medicine practitioners

Complementary practitioners work in some practices in the UK and for certain conditions may have a role to play. For example, yoga and meditation have no side effects and may reduce stress levels and be used a part of the treatment of patients with hypertension, although there is no evidence that they provide any objective benefit.

> It is important that homœopathy and complementary medicine are not advocated as the only treatments offered to patients with serious conditions.

Acupuncture

Many GPs have developed an interest in acupuncture and offer this treatment to patients with various conditions including smoking addiction, musculoskeletal problems, and anxiety. There is no evidence from controlled trials to support the use of acupuncture as a treatment for any cardiovascular risk factor. However, some patients find it helpful and there are no appreciable risks associated with treatment.

Non-clinical staff

Non-clinical staff are crucially important administratively as well as providing their clinical colleagues with moral support and good humour, which is fundamental to an enjoyable working atmosphere.

Reviewing cardiac patients in primary care

GPs are responsible for assessing patients and deciding whether referral to a specialist is appropriate. Appropriate and timely referral is sometimes difficult. A provisional diagnosis is necessary in order to make an appropriate referral. When the diagnosis is clear, the timing of referral requires knowledge of the natural history of the condition, and treatment options. These aspects should be discussed with the patient. Recognising which patients should be referred and when requires experience and judgement and an understanding of their condition. When patients are referred back to the GP after specialist management, it is important for the primary care team to be aware when patients need to be reviewed by a specialist.

The future of primary care as a centre for cardiovascular disease prevention

With sufficient resources and specialist support, primary care clinics should be able to function independently as screening, detection, education and cardiovascular prevention centres for the community. Blood tests, ECGs, stress testing and echocardiography could be performed by trained and accredited GPs and nurses with a special interest in cardiology. Activity, fitness and stress management support and other evolving interventions could be offered near the patients' homes. This should reduce the need for specialist referral. The cost implications are not known.

FURTHER READING

* Luengo-Fernandez R, Leal J, Gray A, Petersen S, Rayner M. Cost of cardiovascular disease in the United Kingdom. *Heart.* 2006; **92:** 1384–9.
* NHS Executive. *National Service Framework for Coronary Heart Disease.* London: Department of Health; 2000.
* Secretary of State for Health. *Saving Lives: our healthier nation.* London: Department of Health; 1999.

Risk factors, risk estimation and use of guidelines

THREE

Risk assessment

An understanding of 'risk' is essential in identifying patients who would benefit from interventions for both primary and secondary prevention as well as those who would not and in whose case treatment is not indicated.

'Risk' is used in several contexts. These include the 'risk' of developing coronary heart disease; the 'risk' of developing a complication from coronary heart disease (for example, myocardial infarction); the 'risk' from an investigation (for example, coronary angiography) or from treatment (medical or surgical). Risk assessment, risk estimation or risk stratification are synonymous and aim to quantify the probability of a condition or clinical event occurring in an individual. Data from clinical, laboratory or other investigations are used to 'quantify' the risk. Some established risk factors are used together with a patient's gender and age to estimate cardiovascular risk.

The risk of cardiovascular disease in populations

Risk assessment data are derived from observing and recording cardiovascular events – angina, myocardial infarction, stroke, death – and monitoring the outcomes in large numbers of patients having a certain condition. The Framingham epidemiology study measures and records cardiovascular risk factors and events among the population living in the town of Framingham, a suburb of Boston, USA. The investigators enrolled more than 5000 residents aged between 30 and 62 years, and examined their progress. In the 1970s, the children of the original cohort of patients joined the study and the project now involves the grandchildren of the original cohort.

Risk factors are not causes

The Framingham study and other long-term epidemiological studies have provided important information on the natural history of cardiovascular disease and the influence of certain conditions – for example, high blood pressure and cholesterol – on morbidity and mortality. Epidemiological studies, in contrast to controlled clinical trials and intervention trials, do not provide information about the effects of treatment. It is also not possible to claim causal relationships between any risk factor and cardiovascular disease. This is why factors linked epidemiologically to cardiovascular disease are referred to as 'risk factors' and not causes.

Risk factors and causes of cardiovascular disease

The presence of a risk factor does not mean that the individual will necessarily develop cardiovascular disease. Conversely, the absence of risk factors does not mean that the individual will *not* develop cardiovascular disease. This is often misunderstood by patients and the bereaved family members of a patient who died from a heart attack and who apparently was perfectly fit and had no risk factors.

When is a condition a risk factor?

A factor is likely to be a risk factor if it fulfils the following criteria.

✧ The association must make clinical sense.

   Clinical observations have often suggested conditions to be risk factors. Some of these appear very simple. In the Framingham study, older people and men under the age of 65 were more likely to die from heart attacks than children and young females. This suggested that increasing age and male gender were risk factors. It was thought that women aged below 65 were less likely than men aged less than 65 to have coronary heart disease. This gender imbalance levels off in later life. Now, for several lifestyle reasons, it is thought that women are at similar risk to men of developing coronary heart disease after the menopause.

✧ Exposure to the proposed risk factor must precede the onset of disease.

✧ The association should make scientific sense.

   The association should be biologically and pathogenetically plausible in animal and clinical studies. It has been known for many years that cholesterol deposits were present in the arteries of animals and people who died from heart attacks and that animals and people with vascular disease were more likely to have a high cholesterol level than those without vascular disease. There must be a strong association between exposure and the incidence of the disease.

✧ The statistical association between the risk factor and cardiovascular disease should be strong.

   Generally, a risk factor should at least double the risk of cardiovascular disease and the association should be dose dependent. For example, the higher the cholesterol or the greater the number of cigarettes smoked, the higher the incidence of cardiovascular disease. This is referred to as a graded relationship.

✧ The risk factor should apply to all populations.

   Framingham was predominantly a white middle-class town shortly after the Second World War. The association between the factors studied and cardiovascular disease applied to all communities of the town and this relationship persisted in subsequent years when the ethnic mix of the town changed. A risk factor should predict consistently cardiovascular disease in a variety of populations. However, some races, for unknown reasons, notably Asians, are at greater risk than Caucasians. Insulin resistance has been proposed to explain this.

✧ Treatment of the risk factor should reduce the risk of cardiovascular disease.

   Statins lower cholesterol levels and reduce cardiovascular risk in both primary and secondary prevention. Treating hypertension also reduces cardiovascular disease.

   Because cardiovascular disease is common and its causes are unknown, it is difficult to prove that treatment for one risk factor lowers cardiovascular risk. This has to be done in a large number of patients in a randomised, placebo-controlled trial. The participants should be representative of the general population and those in whom treatment may be used. There are stages in the natural history of a condition, where it may be too late for an intervention (any treatment or lifestyle modification) to be shown to be effective. Similarly, a very long follow-up and little or no variation in other risk factors would be required in a primary prevention study. In a study evaluating the impact of exercise alone in primary prevention, the result is likely to be difficult to interpret if participants in the non-exercise group changed their diet and lost weight. The apparent effect of exercise in those given an exercise programme may be exaggerated if this group also made a big change to their diet, lowering their cholesterol and weight as well as increasing their daily exercise regime.

✧ The risk factor should exert an independent effect.

It was not clear, until recently, that obesity and lack of physical exercise were independent risk factors.

✧ The risk factor should be measurable.

Stress was suggested for many years to be a risk factor but it is difficult to define and measure. Nevertheless, certain types of stress at work, depression and social isolation are thought to be risk factors. Depression appears to increase risk after myocardial infarction.

Risk factors for coronary heart disease

Most studies have shown that at least 90% of people who died from a myocardial infarction had at least one established cardiovascular risk factor.

TABLE 3.1 Risk factors for coronary heart disease

MODIFIABLE	NON-MODIFIABLE
High LDL	Age
High blood pressure	Gender
Smoking	Family history
Low HDL cholesterol	Genetic
Diabetes and glucose intolerance	
Renal failure	
Birth weight	
Lack of exercise	
Left ventricular hypertrophy	
Central obesity	
Homocysteine	
Clotting factors	
Oral contraceptives	
Stress	
Depression	

The established modifiable and non-modifiable risk factors for coronary heart disease are listed in Table 3.1. The emerging risk factors are discussed in Chapter 4.

TABLE 3.2 Protective factors for coronary heart disease

Moderate alcohol consumption

Exercise

Dietary mono-unsaturates (olive oil, rapeseed oil)

Fruit and vegetables

High HDL cholesterol

Fish oils

Aspirin

Being slim with 'normal' body mass index

Risk assessment and treatment decisions

Risk assessment in cardiovascular disease is the identification of patients with a high or low probability of developing or having coronary heart disease. This is done by estimating a patient's global cardiovascular risk by considering their age and the presence of all their risk factors.

> All adults aged over 40 years and those with a family history of premature coronary disease should have a cardiovascular risk assessment.

Effects of more than one risk factor

The risk posed by individual risk factors is greater in the presence of other risk factors. A high cholesterol level exerts a greater risk if the patient is also diabetic. Dyslipidaemia and diabetes together exert a greater risk if the patient is hypertensive. A person's cardiovascular risk is multiplied several times with the presence of increasing numbers of risk factors.

> A patient with mild elevation of several risk factors may have an unexpectedly high total cardiovascular risk.
> Management of individual risk factors impacts on the total cardiovascular risk.
> A patient's total risk can be reduced even if an individual risk factor (for example, blood pressure control in the elderly) cannot be completely controlled, but the other risk factors are modified.

Which patients should have a cardiovascular risk assessment?

A cardiovascular risk assessment should be performed in patients:

⬧ who are middle-aged (over 40 years of age) and who smoke or have smoked
⬧ with one or more cardiovascular risk factors
⬧ with a family history of vascular disease or a significant risk factor (hypertension, dyslipidaemia)
⬧ with symptoms of vascular disease (angina, transient ischaemic attack, claudication)
⬧ who ask for their risk to be assessed.

> All patients should have lifestyle advice irrespective of their estimated risk.

Who is at high risk?

Patients with the following conditions and risk factors should be treated with lifestyle modifications and tablets as necessary:

⬧ established vascular disease (angina, myocardial infarction, cerebrovascular disease, stroke)
⬧ diabetes
⬧ smoking
⬧ obesity
⬧ renal disease with eGFR of <60 mL/min/1.73 m^2
⬧ those with a >20% 10-year risk of developing cardiovascular disease (European Society of Cardiology Guidelines recommend using drugs as part of the treatment for patients with a SCORE risk of >5%)
⬧ elevated blood pressure with systolic >160/100 mmHg and/or diastolic >100 mmHg, or lower levels but with end organ damage
⬧ elevated total cholesterol : HDL cholesterol ratio of >6.0
⬧ familial dyslipidaemia
⬧ family history of premature cardiovascular disease.

> High-risk patients have:
> ● vascular disease
> ● type 2 diabetes or type 1 diabetes with microalbuminuria
> ● high levels of individual risk factors.

Who is at low risk?

The following characteristics identify healthy people at low risk:

⬧ never smoked
⬧ total cholesterol <5 mol/L, LDL cholesterol <3 mol/L and glucose <6 mmol/l

✧   exercise every day for 30 minutes
✧   slim
✧   healthy diet
✧   normal renal function
✧   normal glucose level
✧   no family history of premature coronary heart disease
✧   blood pressure <140/85 mmHg.

Aims of cardiovascular prevention

> The aims of cardiovascular prevention are to improve quality of life, reduce cardio-
> vascular mortality, reduce the risk of cardiovascular disease and its complications,
> and the need for revascularisation.

Establishing a rapport with the patient

Effective prevention depends on the clinician having a good rapport with the patient. In order for patients to make meaningful changes to their lifestyle, they must understand the concept of risk factors, the risks of not changing their lifestyle, the benefits of risk factor reduction, and what they need to do in order to reduce their risk. Long-term patient education, risk factor evaluation, monitoring and support are the cornerstones of prevention.

The clinician has to understand the personal and domestic components which patients consider practical impediments to change. Some risk factors can be modified or treated with lifestyle modifications or treatments: diet, exercise, smoking, hypertension and diabetes. Others, such as work-related stress, financial pressures, or personal or marital relationships, are more difficult for the clinician to modify. Practical advice and support can be offered, but only after all these components have been identified. Patients may be unwilling to discuss certain issues.

Setting agreed achievable objectives is important. Giving the patient easily understood dietary advice and agreeing a target weight for the next consultation gives the patient a clear goal. Subsequent consultations provide the opportunity for reinforcement of the prevention message. Effective prevention and lifestyle modification requires frequent consultations.

The way this advice is given should be tailored to the patient.

Difficulties with prevention strategies

Initiating and ensuring long-term patient compliance with cardiovascular prevention is practically difficult. Effective management of this important but time-consuming work depends on good practice organisation and the knowledge, enthusiasm, skill and commitment of staff aware of the difficulties of persuading patients to change their day-to-day lives by stopping life-long pleasurable habits and taking tablets for the rest of their lives. Patients make these sacrifices in return for the possibility of living longer with a lower risk of developing a stroke, heart attack, heart failure or renal failure. Lifestyle modification is more difficult in younger patients who generally have a less acute sense of their own mortality.

With an aging and diverse population, this task is not getting easier because the potential benefits are not immediately apparent to either the patient or clinician. It is not surprising that even with the skills of dedicated staff, patients find it very difficult to maintain long-term lifestyle changes. The following factors may account for this:

- reluctance to give up pleasurable habits
- low socio-economic class, low educational level, low income
- social isolation, particularly in the elderly
- depression, anxiety and doubt about the value of lifestyle changes
- conflicting or confusing advice.

Clinical and laboratory information

The following information from the history, examination and laboratory tests are important for a comprehensive risk assessment.

History

- Ethnicity.
- Symptoms of angina, previous infarction, transient ischaemic attack or stroke, claudication.
- Smoking.
- Exercise.
- Diet.
- Family history of cardiovascular disease.

Examination

- Blood pressure.
- Cardiac examination.
- Foot pulses.
- Aortic aneurysm.
- Carotid bruits.
- Height, weight, waist circumference.
- Signs of dyslipidaemia (xanthomata, xanthelasma).

Laboratory tests

- Urine dipstix and urinalysis if there is glucose, blood, protein, microalbuminuria.
- Lipids including LDL cholesterol (fasting simplifies the problem of raised levels).
- Glucose, renal function.

Cardiac investigations

The need for these depend on the clinical features found.

✧ ECG.

✧ Exercise test.

✧ Echocardiogram for patients with hypertension or murmurs.

Deciding when to treat

Knowledge of the natural history of the condition is essential. It is important to understand the aims for drug treatment. For example, deciding to use drug treatments to improve prognosis in a 90-year-old has much less clinical relevance than the same decision in the case of a 60-year-old. However, the 90-year-old is at greater risk and drug treatments are likely to exert a greater benefit in those at greater risk.

Treatment decisions are based on the patient's global risk and a judgement of the benefits and risks of treatment against the risks of non-treatment. Treatment decisions are influenced by practical and financial considerations.

Treatment decisions are difficult when data from trials do not translate to the patient sitting in front of you. This is most commonly encountered in the elderly who are usually excluded from controlled clinical trials.

Coronary vs cardiovascular disease risk

Currently available risk-factor tools estimate a patient's *coronary heart disease* risk using the patient's age, gender, smoking habit, systolic blood pressure, the presence of diabetes and whether the patient has known vascular disease and target organ damage. *Cardiovascular disease risk*, which includes the risk of stroke, is calculated by multiplying the coronary heart disease risk by 4/3. Thus, a patient with a coronary heart disease risk of 30% has a cardiovascular disease risk of 40%. This conversion is less accurate at the extremes of age.

Global cardiovascular risk

Total cardiovascular risk, rather than coronary risk, should be estimated because atheromatous vascular disease affects cerebral, carotid, renal and peripheral arteries, not only coronary arteries.

Most clinicians in the UK use the Joint British Societies' cardiovascular risk prediction charts. These incorporate only age, gender, smoking habit, systolic blood pressure and the ratio of total cholesterol : HDL cholesterol, and whether the patient is diabetic.

The SCORE charts estimate total cardiovascular risk and are used in Europe. The Framingham risk score, devised in 1967, was the first risk chart and an updated version is used in the USA.

A patient's absolute or overall cardiovascular risk is estimated from risk charts. If the 10-year risk is >20% the individual is at high risk and treatment is appropriate.

Influence of age on risk estimation: relative risk vs absolute risk

Most men over 50 and most women over 60 have a 20% or greater risk of developing cardiovascular disease. Most young people, despite the presence of important risk factors, would be categorised at low absolute risk and therefore would not reach the somewhat arbitrary threshold for drug treatments.

Relative risk is a clinically more meaningful concept than absolute risk in young patients. Relative risk can be estimated using the European Society of Guidelines Relative Risk Chart. Even with several risk factors, young people would have a low 10-year absolute cardiovascular risk. Compared with people of the same age, however, their relative risk is high. Young patients with one or more cardiovascular risk factors may have a low absolute cardiovascular risk that falls below the treatment threshold simply because they are young. Treatment should not be discounted in younger patients solely on this basis and the decision to use drugs, as in the elderly, should be carefully considered and discussed with the patient. Explaining relative risk to young patients may help them decide about switching to a healthy lifestyle. Young patients with a high relative risk who are not treated initially should be monitored and may need drug treatments later.

Absolute risk

A patient's absolute risk of developing cardiovascular disease associated with exposure to a condition, for example, hypertension, is the rate of development of new cases of disease per unit of time. The development of new cases of disease per unit time is the incidence of disease.

Absolute risk also determines the probability of benefit from antihypertensive treatment. Treatment guidelines for hypertension and hyperlipidaemia are based on absolute risk estimation which is composed by weighting appropriately all the major risk factors.

Absolute risk reduction

Using the example of a randomised, placebo-controlled trial, the *absolute risk reduction* is the difference in the probabilities of an event in the control and treatment groups. If the adverse event rate in the treatment group is less than in the control group, this indicates a potential benefit from the treatment.

Relative risk

The relative risk of disease is the ratio of disease incidence among exposed individuals compared to non-exposed individuals. Therefore, relative risk measures the strength of the association between exposure and disease. Relative risk may suggest causality but it gives no indication of the absolute risk of disease.

The relative benefit of an active treatment over a control is usually expressed as the *relative risk*, the relative risk reduction or the odds ratio. It is used to characterise the relative effect of a treatment in a group of patients compared with a placebo and not to individual patients. In a controlled randomised trial, for example, the relative risk of the treatment is the probability of an event in the active treatment group divided by the probability of an event in the control group. Beneficial treatments would have a relative risk of less than one.

Relative risk reduction

The relative risk reduction is derived by subtracting the relative risk from 1. Therefore, a relative risk of 0 indicates that the treatment results in neither benefit no harm. Relative risk reduction can also be expressed as absolute reduction divided by the probability of an event in the control arm.

Relative risk reduction does not translate to individual benefit

Hypertension treatment decreases the risk of all cardiovascular complications by around 25% mainly by reducing stroke by 38% and coronary events by 16%. The *relative risk reduction* of antihypertensive treatment is 25% in all groups of patients – male and females of all ages, and smokers and non-smokers. However, the chance that an individual patient will benefit from antihypertensive treatment depends on their absolute risk from a cardiovascular complication. The estimated relative risk reduction of 25% may apply to those patients at moderate to high risk of a cardiovascular complication but not to patients at low risk and so the potential toxicity and cost of the treatment may outweigh its small potential benefits.

Absolute risk reduction and the 'number needed to treat'

This is the number of patients a clinician needs to treat with a particular drug to expect to prevent one adverse event. It can be expressed as the *reciprocal of the absolute risk reduction*. In clinical decision-making, it is useful and meaningful to use the term 'number needed to treat' because it enables clinicians and patients to think of treatment benefits in terms of patients and not abstract probabilities. It is calculated as the inverse of the absolute risk reduction.

For example, a group of patients with untreated *moderate* hypertension has a 20% *absolute risk* of stroke but this is reduced to 12% with antihypertensive treatment which confers a *relative risk reduction* of 40%. The *absolute risk reduction* is 0.20 − 0.12 = 0.08. The reciprocal of this number is 13, implying that the clinician would *need to treat around 13 moderately hypertensive patients* for five years before preventing one stroke.

In contrast, consider a group of patients with untreated *mild* hypertension with a 15% *absolute risk* of stroke but this is reduced to 9% with antihypertensive treatment which confers a *relative risk reduction* of 40%. The absolute risk reduction is 0.15 − 0.9 = 0.6. The reciprocal of this number is 167. Therefore, the clinician would need to treat 167 patients with *mild hypertension* for five years to expect to prevent one stroke. These examples are useful for clinicians and can be used to explain management decisions to patients who may be confused about the advice they are given which depends on their absolute risk and the estimated absolute risk reduction.

TABLE 3.3 Absolute and relative cardiovascular risk estimation and numbers needed to treat

	PATIENT A	PATIENT B
Blood pressure	165/100	165/100
Gender	Male	Female
Age	60	44
Diabetes	yes	no
Total : HDL cholesterol	8	4
Smoker	yes	no
Left ventricular hypertrophy	yes	no
Family history of infarction	yes	yes
Absolute 10-year CHD risk	60%	<2%
Relative risk reduction	40%	40%
Absolute benefit	24%	0.8%
Number needed to treat (for 5 years)	4	125

Table 3.3 provides another example using 10-year absolute coronary heart disease risk derived from the Joint British Societies' Risk Prediction Chart. It can be seen that the absolute benefit of treating these two patients depends largely on their baseline absolute risk. The number of patients needed to be treated for five years to prevent one stroke is correspondingly very different; four patients with the absolute risk characterised by patient A and 125 patients with the absolute risk of patient B. Therefore, before recommending long-term, costly treatment that may have adverse effects, the decision to treat a hypertensive patient should be based on their absolute risk and not simply on their blood-pressure reading.

Risk prevention tables and charts

There are several tools to estimate coronary heart disease risk and most are based on the Framingham data, which is the only published epidemiological study in which both men and women are included.

Framingham risk equations

These were developed to predict the 10-year risk of coronary heart disease, heart failure or stroke and the average risk in age- and sex-matched controls. The subjects from Boston, Massachusetts, were mainly white, middle-class people. This is important because certain high-risk groups, for example, South Indian Asians, were not included. A reasonable but, by current standards, incomplete range of risk factors was measured. For example, family history, inactivity and obesity were not included and the protective influence of high HDL levels and the high risk of high LDL levels were not appreciated at the time. It is difficult, however, to include all emerging or potential risk factors in a risk assessment table until they have been validated and so this criticism could be applied in retrospect to any risk estimation tool.

Dundee coronary risk disk

This provides an estimate of a person's relative risk for coronary mortality matched for age and sex. It was derived in men only and has not been independently validated in women and may not be applicable to other populations. It does not correlate very well to Framingham estimates.

British Regional Heart Study risk function

This has not been independently validated and cannot be used to predict risk in women, and may underestimate risk.

The predictive accuracy of any risk factor assessment system depends on the inclusion of all relevant prognostic information. This should include data from a large study population including people of different ethnicity so that the information is representative of the population to whom the results will be applied. These tools also require updating to include newly established risk factors and should take account of protective risk factors.

Comparison of different risk charts and tables

There are several different risk charts. The European Society of Cardiology has risk charts for high- and low-risk areas of Europe reflecting the wide geographical area and lifestyles of north and south Europe. The Joint British Societies' (British Cardiac Society, British Diabetic Society and British Hyperlipidaemia Society) risk chart is probably the most accurate. The Sheffield table, the New Zealand Charts and the European charts are less accurate in coronary risk prevention. There is a computer programme available from the British Heart Foundation.

The Joint British Societies' risk chart incorporates gender, age, smoking status, systolic blood pressure, and total : HDL cholesterol ratio. The chart is relatively easy to use and accurate. The limitations are the non-inclusion of other important risk factors (*see* Tables 3.1 and 3.2). The classification for smoking of 'yes/no' does not differentiate between a person who stopped smoking 60 cigarettes a day the week before and a person who has never smoked. Diabetic patients are assessed using a separate chart, which is illogical as they are at high risk and should be treated.

Young people may be under-treated because they do not reach the risk treatment threshold of 30%. For example, the current guidelines would not recommend treating a 30-year-old diabetic, hypertensive, female smoker with high cholesterol. Treatment for old men would be recommended, however, in view of age and gender.

The Joint British Societies' computerised risk assessment differs from the chart by incorporating diastolic blood pressure, serum cholesterol, HDL cholesterol, diabetes (yes/no) and left ventricular hypertrophy on electrocardiogram (yes/no) as well as age, gender and systolic blood pressure. It has similar limitations to the chart because variables like smoking and blood sugar, which confer an incremental risk are scored categorically as either 'yes' or 'no'.

Using risk-prevention tables and charts in primary care is not easy but may become so with user-friendly desktop computer programmes and the availability of straightforward, up-to-date, comprehensive systems that integrate with patients' clinical data. Importantly, the risk-assessment programme should be based on clinical data and therefore applicable to the patients treated in the practice where the programme is to be used. Other information showing the differential weighting of risk factors and the potential incremental and total benefits of modifying each one would be helpful. This type of programme could provide risk assessment relevant to the patient in front of you, audit facilities and graphic illustrations. It would also provide an interactive capability to allow patients to understand, participate in and take the principal role in their own self-administered and motivated cardiovascular risk management.

> Calculating cardiovascular risk to help decide treatment strategies in individual patients is of value only if the patient takes the treatment and makes other synergistic long-term lifestyle changes.

General practitioners and practice nurses are able to evaluate the risk of coronary heart disease with only moderate accuracy because not all the required risk factors, for example HDL cholesterol levels, may be available in the patients' records.

Different experts, different views

The majority of patients will not need specialist referral and will be managed in primary care using risk tables and charts to guide treatment strategies for individual patients. Hypertension, hyperlipidaemia or diabetes may be diagnosed only when patients are admitted to hospital with a myocardial infarction or stroke or other cardiovascular problem. Treatment for these risk factors may be started in hospital or recommendations may be made for the general practitioner to decide whether treatment is necessary after discharge.

> Patients may have seen different specialists with different opinions. The primary care team will have to consider all the advice which may differ.
>
> It is helpful for all clinicians running prevention clinics for the same patient population to give consistent and uniform advice to reduce confusion among patients. Short prevention pamphlets written in accessible English, or the language the patient prefers, are useful.

The role of the primary care team

Risk-factor reduction clinics are now usually run by nurses in primary care. Patients should be educated about absolute cardiovascular risk and take responsibility for improving their risk profile with continual encouragement and monitoring. All risk factors should be discussed. Patients should understand their crucial role in their long-term health and what changes they may need to make to their lifestyle.

The primary care team is uniquely placed to assess cardiovascular risk and initiate, monitor and review interventions to improve a patient's long-term risk profile with a view to lowering their risk of cardiovascular events. In patients with established atheromatous vascular disease and referred for specialist care, this may be done in conjunction with a variety of hospital staff including cardiologists, diabetologists, hypertension specialists, cardiac nurse specialists, pharmacists and rehabilitation team members. The long-term responsibility and burden of management will fall on those working in primary care.

Role of nurses

Nurses are playing an increasingly important role in risk-factor management and are key members of the primary care team. Nurse-managed programmes have been shown to be effective in the management of single risk factors including diet, smoking cessation, lipid lowering, diabetes and hypertension. They now run comprehensive risk-factor modification and rehabilitation clinics.

Management protocols and teaching and training courses on these subjects have provided nurses with the necessary skills and experience to identify patients who may benefit from drug interventions and need specialist referral. These include patients who are resistant to treatment, those at high risk or those who want a specialist opinion.

Variations in coronary heart disease incidence and outcomes

There are well-recognised variations in cardiovascular disease outcomes in Britain with comparatively high mortality rates in Scotland and some parts of northern England. The causes of this are unclear but may be due to cultural, socio-economic, age and lifestyle differences.

Diet is an important influence on cholesterol levels, particularly LDL cholesterol and coronary heart disease mortality. The low LDL cholesterol levels in rural Japanese and Chinese people probably explain their low myocardial infarction rates despite their high rates of smoking. People with a low LDL cholesterol level have a very low risk of acute vascular events.

Variations in secondary care management of coronary heart disease

Local variations in coronary heart disease morbidity and mortality are more difficult to measure but clinicians may be aware of organisational arrangements where patients with acute presentations of coronary heart disease may be seen by non-cardiologists and would be less likely to have invasive investigation and intervention. Management protocols can only be effective if they are applied. This depends on the clinical team making the correct diagnosis. Local variations in practice between cardiologists may also affect outcomes. Cardiologists trained in interventional techniques are more likely than non-interventionists to recommend an invasive and interventional strategy to patients with coronary artery syndromes. Patients admitted to a hospital with comprehensive cardiology and cardiac surgical facilities are more likely to have coronary angiography and myocardial revascularisation than patients admitted to a hospital without these facilities.

Specialists may have a different view of the importance of risk factors and advocate investigations or treatments not recommended in local guidelines. Some cardiologists, for example, test for and treat high homocysteine levels with folic acid. Cardiologists vary in their attitude and approach to weight loss, diet and exercise. Some, for a number of reasons, leave risk management to their colleagues in primary care.

Legal implications of guidelines in clinical management

A guideline may be defined as information designed to aid a practitioner and patient to pursue the most appropriate healthcare response to specific clinical circumstances. They are usually based on scientific evidence.

Clinicians may be concerned about the legal implications of deviating from guidelines and whether adherence to guidelines protects them from liability.

In UK law:

> the mere fact that a protocol or guideline exists for the care of a particular condition does not of itself establish that compliance with it would be reasonable in the circumstances, or that non-compliance would be negligent. As guideline-informed health care increasingly becomes customary, so acting outside the guidance of guidelines could expose doctors to the possibility of being found negligent, unless they can prove a special justification in the circumstances.

> Guidelines are guidelines, not law. They have to be applied according to the patient's specific clinical circumstances taking account of the clinician's considered view, the opinion of his colleagues when applicable, the patient's wishes and logistic, practical and economic factors.

Clinical management guidelines are relatively new and are being formulated for an increasing number of procedures and conditions. They are consensus statements based on available data from clinical trials with specified, acceptable protocol characteristics, including double-blind treatments, adequate follow-up, randomisation to either active or placebo treatments, appropriate and balanced patient demography, 'hard' end-points relevant to the question asked of the trial and adequate statistical power. It is important to remember that the interpretation of trial results is based on opinion and that guidelines are not infallible.

Treatment guidelines for coronary heart disease are based on estimated *absolute coronary heart disease risk*. They are designed to help clinicians, patients and others involved in funding healthcare, make informed and appropriate clinical decisions and to reduce healthcare costs. They have benefits and drawbacks (*see* Tables 3.1 and 3.2).

Abba Eban, the former Israeli Ambassador to the United Nations said 'consensus means that lots of people say collectively what no one believes individually'. Nevertheless, guidelines are here to stay and if used wisely, can enhance, simplify and standardise clinical management. They do not, however, remove the need for sound, experienced clinical judgement and should not displace a critical and questioning attitude. Ultimately, the clinician responsible for the care of the patient has to decide whether the guidelines proposed are relevant and should be applied to the patient sitting in the consulting room.

Potential benefits of guidelines
- Ensure a minimum quality of care.
- Standardise management of high-volume, procedure-related activities and common clinical conditions.
- Reduce the use of inappropriate or unproven investigations or treatment.
- Provide comparative procedural outcome data for audit.
- Push up clinical quality of 'average' institutions to the 'best'.
- Restrict the use of costly procedures or treatments to situations where there is sufficient evidence that they are 'effective'.

Potential drawbacks of guidelines
- Interpretation of trial results is based on opinion.
- The guideline writers may not be active clinicians in the relevant field.
- Randomised trials usually include only low-risk individuals and the results may not be relevant to the patient in the real world, for whom other clinical considerations and their personal wishes demand individualised management.
- Ensure only a minimum quality of care.
- Decisions based on cost and consensus may deprive patients of new treatments.
- Loss of professional autonomy.
- Stifle creativity and innovation – 'cookbook medicine'.
- Lead to mediocre rather than high-quality medicine.
- Guidelines may not be applicable to individual patients.
- May be out of date or redundant.
- Litigation concerns.
- The condition or disease may change.

Value, use and limitations of guidelines
Examples of guidelines leading to organisational changes and improved clinical outcomes include reduction in door-to-needle times and the secondary prevention treatments after myocardial infarction.

Guideline utilisation is increased if the guidelines make clinical sense, are clear, concise and up to date, and apply to the overwhelming majority of patients with the specified condition. One current major problem is the large number of guidelines from a variety of sources (local and national) for the same condition. Clinicians find this confusing and overwhelming and this may make them disinclined to use any of them.

Advice for patients

✧ Your risk of developing heart disease depends on a number of risk factors. These are not the same as causes but increase the chances of you developing furring up of the heart and other arteries.

✧ People who have risk factors may or may not need tablets. The decision is made by estimating your risk based on your age and other factors, for example, your blood pressure and cholesterol level. This means that even though you may have a friend who is not taking tablets, you need them because you are at greater risk of developing heart disease because of you have risk factors that they don't have.

FURTHER READING

Anderson KM, Odell PM, Wilson PWF, et al. Cardiovascular disease risk profiles. Am Heart J. 1990; **121:** 293–8.

Armstrong PW. Do guidelines influence practice? Heart. 2003; **89:** 349–52.

British Cardiac Society, British Hyperlipidaemia Association, British Hypertension Society, British Diabetic Association. Joint British recommendations on prevention of coronary heart disease in clinical practice: summary. BMJ. 2000; **320:** 705–8.

Cook RJ, Sackett DL. The number needed to treat: a clinically useful measure of treatment effect. BMJ. 1995; **310:** 452–4.

Department of Health. National Service Framework for Coronary Heart Disease. London: Department of Health, 2000.

Durrington PN, Prais H, Bhatnagar D, et al. Indications for cholesterol-lowering medication: comparison of risk-assessment methods. Lancet. 1999; **353:** 278–81.

Grimshaw JM, Russell IT. Effect of clinical guidelines on medical practice: a systematic review of rigorous evaluations. Lancet. 1993; **342:** 1317–22.

Hampton JR. Guidelines – for the obedience of fools and the guidance of wise men? Clin Med. 2003; **3:** 279–84.

Jones AF, Walker J, Jewkes C, et al. Comparative accuracy of cardiovascular risk prediction methods in primary care patients. Heart. 2001; **85:** 37–43.

McManus RJ, Mant J, Meulendijks CF, et al. Comparison of estimates and calculations of risk of coronary heart disease by doctors and nurses using different calculation tools in general practice: cross-sectional study. BMJ. 2002; **324:** 459–64.

Nash IS. Practice guidelines in cardiovascular care. In: Fuster V, Alexander RW, O'Rourke RA, editors. Hurst's 'The Heart', 10th ed. New York: McGraw Hill; 2001.

National Cholesterol Education Program. Executive summary of the third report of the National Cholesterol Education Program (NCEP) expert panel on detection, evaluation, and treatment of high blood cholesterol in adults (adult treatment panel III). JAMA. 2001; **285:** 2486–97.

Poulter N. Global risk of cardiovascular disease. Heart. 2003; **89(Suppl):** 2ii.

Shaper AG, Pocock SJ, Phillips AN, Walker M. Identifying men at high risk of heart attacks: strategy for use in general practice. BMJ. 1986; **293:** 474–9.

Tunstall-Pedoe H. The Dundee coronary risk-disk for management of change in risk factors. 1991; **303:** 744–7.

Wilson PW, D'Agostino R, Levy D, et al. Prediction of coronary heart disease using risk factor categories. Circulation. 1998; **97:** 1837–47.

Wolf PA, D'Agostino RB, Belanger AJ, Silbershatz H, Kannel WB. Probability of stroke: a risk profile from the Framingham study. *Stroke.* 1991; **22:** 312–18.

Wolf PA, D'Agostino RB, Silbershatz H, Belanger AJ, Wilson PWF, Levy D. Profile for estimating risk of heart failure. *Arch Intern Med.* 1999; **159:** 1197–1204.

Wood D, De Backer G, Faergeman O, *et al.*, with members of the Task Force. Prevention of coronary heart disease in clinical practice: recommendations of the second joint task force of European and other societies on coronary prevention. *Atherosclerosis.* 1998; **140:** 199–270

Wood D, Durrington PN, Poulter N, *et al.* Joint British recommendations on prevention of coronary heart disease in clinical practice. *Heart.* 1998; **80(Suppl 2):** S1–29.

Legal implications of guidelines

Schwartz PJ, Breithard G, Howard AJ, *et al.* The legal implications of medical guidelines – a Task Force of the European Society of Cardiology. *Eur Heart J.* 1999; **20:** 1152–7.

Hypertension

FOUR

Clinical cases

1. A 40-year-old symptom-free man who is moderately overweight has a blood sugar level of 7 mmol/l and is worried about his blood pressure, which he checks himself frequently and he records as 150/100 mmHg. What do you do?
2. A 75-year-old known hypertensive man comes to see you with headache, and you record his blood pressure as 190/150 mmHg. What do you do?
3. A 34-year-old woman is 28 weeks into her second pregnancy, having been diagnosed as having borderline hypertension during her first uncomplicated pregnancy four years ago. She feels well, but the nurse in the hospital antenatal clinic found her blood pressure to be 145/95 mmHg. What do you do?
4. A fit 86-year-old woman has a blood pressure of 175/80 mmHg but, because she feels fine, can do the crossword and does a lot of voluntary work at the old-age home, is not keen to take any tablets. What do you advise her to do?
5. A 67-year-old obese woman with type 2 diabetes, hyperlipidaemia and mild claudication has a blood pressure of 165/95 mmHg, despite taking a thiazide diuretic and an angiotensin-converting-enzyme inhibitor. How do you manage her?
6. A 74-year-old man with a history of myocardial infarction and stroke has been taking a β-blocker for his hypertension for more than 20 years. His blood pressure is well controlled. Should he remain on the β-blocker?

The public health implications of hypertension

The World Health Organization has ranked hypertension as the most important cause of death worldwide. The screening for hypertension and its continual monitoring, treatment and control, as part of a comprehensive or global strategy of cardiovascular prevention, constitutes a major part of the workload in primary care. Good hypertension management makes an important difference to the health of the individual, and a well-organised hypertension clinic reduces cardiovascular disease in the population.

Definitions and classification of hypertension

Hypertension is graded in three categories, as shown in Table 4.1.

Hypertension is defined as a systolic blood pressure of >140 mmHg and/or a diastolic pressure of >85 mmHg. Optimal blood pressure is defined as <120/80 mmHg. Isolated systolic hypertension is a systolic pressure of >140 mmHg and a diastolic pressure of <90 mmHg.

TABLE 4.1 Classification of blood pressure

CATEGORY	SYSTOLIC (MMHG)	DIASTOLIC (MMHG)
Optimal	<120 and	<80
Normal	120–129 and/or	80–84
High normal	130–139 and/or	85–89
Grade 1 hypertension	140–159 and/or	90–99
Grade 2 hypertension	160–179 and/or	100–109
Grade 3 hypertension	>180 and/or	>110
Isolated systolic hypertension	>140 and	<90

Systolic and diastolic pressures are prognostically equally important, although some studies have shown a stronger relationship between hypertension and stroke than between hypertension and coronary events.

There is a graded independent relationship between systolic and diastolic pressure with heart failure, peripheral artery disease and end-stage renal disease.

Current issues in hypertension

✧ The cause of hypertension is unknown in more than 90% of patients.

✧ Hypertension remains under-diagnosed. Many patients with 'mild' hypertension are untreated, and the majority of those with 'severe' hypertension are under-treated or not taking the prescribed medication. Thus, large numbers of people who do not regularly see their GP (notably middle-aged men) are at unnecessarily high risk of coronary heart disease and stroke.

✧ Fewer than 10% of hypertensive patients are controlled at 'target' levels.

✧ There is a reluctance to treat elderly patients with 'mild hypertension' and isolated systolic hypertension.

✧ White-coat hypertension is recognised by clinicians and patients, but its prognostic implications and the need for treatment remain unclear.

✧ The roles of ambulatory blood pressure recordings and self-monitored recordings as useful diagnostic and monitoring tools, and their use and place in diagnosis and treatment, are becoming clearer. They are recommended to provide a more comprehensive view of a patient's blood pressure. High home recordings may be due to anxiety but not 'white-coat syndrome'. The readings still need careful interpretation.

✧ β-blockers are less effective than other classes of antihypertensive drugs in reducing major cardiovascular events (particularly stroke) and diabetes. They are no longer recommended as either first- or second-line medication unless there are good clinical reasons for using them (e.g. angina, previous infarction).

✧ Most patients with hypertension will require more than one type of drug to reduce their blood pressure to the target level.

✧ Combination treatment as initial therapy is not yet recommended, but would probably be more effective than initial treatment with a single drug.

✧ Consensus guidelines have recommended lower target blood pressure levels for patients with a high absolute cardiovascular risk, including diabetics, smokers and those with coronary artery disease or target organ damage, particularly left ventricular hypertrophy. It is important that these groups of high-risk patients are identified and treated effectively.

✧ Compliance with drug and non-pharmacological treatment can be improved by explaining to patients the nature of hypertension, its complications and potential drug side effects, and by continual clinical monitoring and checks on tablet intake. Once-daily dosing improves compliance.

Hypertension as a primary care specialty

The vast majority of patients with hypertension are diagnosed, treated and monitored within primary care. Patients with suspected secondary hypertension and who may need further complex investigations, individuals with important postural hypotension and those whose blood pressure is not adequately controlled need referral to hospital. Pregnant women with hypertension should be referred for a specialist opinion, although this would be detected during antenatal checks. Accelerated or malignant hypertension is now rarely seen, and these patients should be referred to hospital for urgent assessment and treatment.

Tasks for primary care clinicians in managing hypertension

✧ Identify people with hypertension.
✧ Establish blood pressure values.
✧ Identify people with secondary hypertension.
✧ Evaluate the total cardiovascular risk.
✧ Look for end-organ damage and complications.
✧ Look for other diseases.
✧ Carry out at least annual monitoring of blood pressure and response to medication. Young patients may need less frequent evaluation.
✧ Start the most appropriate medication.
✧ Plan and explain long-term management.

Recording the history in a patient with hypertension

This information can be obtained by asking the patient to fill in a tick-box history sheet. The data can then be entered into their computerised records.

1. *Duration and previous level of blood pressure.* Women should be asked about hypertension during pregnancy.

2. *Clues to possible secondary hypertension:*
✧ family history of renal disease due to polycystic kidney disease

✧ renal disease, urinary tract infection, haematuria, analgesic abuse causing renal paren-chymal disease
✧ drugs/illicit substances – oral contraceptives, liquorice, carbenoxolone, cocaine, amphetamines, steroids, non-steroidal anti-inflammatory drugs, cyclosporin
✧ sweating, headache, anxiety, palpitation – phaeochromocytoma
✧ muscle weakness and tetany – aldosteronism.

3. *Cardiovascular risk factors*:
✧ family history of hypertension and cardiovascular disease
✧ family and personal history of dyslipidaemia
✧ family and personal history of diabetes
✧ smoking
✧ dietary habits
✧ obesity
✧ exercise habits
✧ snoring and sleep apnoea
✧ stress.

4. *Clinical features of cardiovascular disease*:
✧ angina, heart failure, carotid bruits, fundal examination (haemorrhages, exudates and papilloedema are now rarely seen in modern practice)
✧ transient ischaemic attacks
✧ claudication (radio-femoral delay, decreased foot pulses)
✧ waist measurement and weight.

Routine investigations in hypertensive patients

Sub-clinical organ damage is a bad prognostic sign.

TABLE 4.2 Routine tests in hypertensive patients

TEST	CLINICAL INDICATION
ECG	Left ventricular hypertrophy, ischaemia, infarction
Echocardiography	Heart murmurs or hypertension, left ventricular hypertrophy
Carotid ultrasound	Carotid bruits or a history of transient ischaemic attacks
Renal function[a]	Creatinine clearance, eGFR, urinary protein by dipstix
Spot urine[b]	Microalbuminuria, relate to urinary creatinine if dipstix is negative
Quantitative proteinuria	If dipstix is positive, measure albumin excretion
Ankle-brachial index	Claudication or reduced leg pulses
Glucose tolerance test	If fasting glucose level is >5.6 mmol/l (100 mg/dl)
Home and 24-hour BP recording	Suspected white coat syndrome, episodic symptoms

a Hypertension-induced kidney damage is shown by reduced renal function and/or increased excretion of albumin. The estimated glomerular filtration rate (eGFR) is calculated using the patient's age, gender, race and serum creatinine concentration. There are two methods of estimating the eGFR, both of which identify

patients with renal disease even if the creatinine level remains normal. Values below 60 ml/min/1.73 m²
indicate chronic renal disease stage 3.

b Urinary protein should be measured with a dipstick. In both hypertensive and diabetic patients, microalbuminuria is associated with increased cardiovascular disease.

Tests are done to determine whether there is left ventricular hypertrophy, diastolic
dysfunction, atherosclerotic vascular disease or kidney damage, all of which put the
patient in a poor prognostic group, and necessitate vigorous risk-factor modification.
The tests listed in Table 4.2 are widely available and are cost-effective.

Haemodynamic changes in hypertension

Hypertension occurs when excessive vasoconstriction and/or volume are not compensated
by adequate pressure natriuresis or suppression of the renin–aldosterone system.

Hypertension and pulse pressure as cardiovascular risk factors: benefits of lowering blood pressure

Hypertension is the most common cause of stroke, the most common reversible
cause of heart failure and an important cause of coronary heart disease (particularly
in diabetics) and renal disease. The relationship between blood pressure and
cardiovascular disease is continuous and graded, and there is no cut-off value that
separates those patients who will and those who will not develop a cardiovascular
event.

The risk of an individual developing cardiovascular disease depends on the level of the
blood pressure and coexisting risk factors. Because hypertension and other risk factors
are common, most hypertensive patients have other risk factors and also sub-clinical
organ damage. Risk is directly proportional to systolic blood pressure and inversely
proportional to diastolic blood pressure.

Isolated systolic hypertension is defined as a systolic blood pressure of ≥140 mmHg and a
diastolic pressure of <90 mmHg. It is the most common form of hypertension, occurring
in over two-thirds of people over 65 years and three-quarters of those over 75 years of age.
In patients over 50 years of age, elevation of systolic blood pressure predicts the risk of
stroke better than increases in diastolic blood pressure. Lowering systolic blood pressure
to <150 mmHg is associated with reductions of 40% in stroke, 16% in coronary events,
50% in heart failure and 15% in mortality.

In patients under 50 years of age, diastolic blood pressure is a stronger predictor of
fatal and non-fatal coronary artery disease. Above the age of 60 years diastolic pressure is
inversely related to coronary risk so that *pulse pressure* (systolic pressure minus diastolic
pressure) is a better predictor of cardiovascular events than systolic blood pressure.

The increasing systolic blood pressure increases left ventricular work and the risk of hypertrophy. The lowering of the diastolic blood pressure compromises coronary blood flow. Thus a blood pressure of 150/85 mmHg carries a higher risk than does a blood pressure of 150/95 mmHg in patients over 60 years of age. A wide pulse pressure is an important risk factor, and lowering of the systolic blood pressure alone is a primary objective of treating hypertension, but difficult to achieve. Pulse pressure is also highly predictive of cardiovascular risk. This is because the higher the pulse pressure, the greater the pressure stress on arterial walls, and the more likely it is that there will be organ damage. A blood pressure recording of 150/95 mmHg has different implications for a 70-year-old man than for a 35-year-old man. The 70-year-old man has a higher absolute cardiovascular risk, but the 35-year-old man has a higher relative risk compared with 'normal' men of his age.

Observational studies suggest that the lower the blood pressure the better – although this notion is not confirmed by individual outcome trials, except in diabetics.

New epidemiological and clinical trial data have reshaped treatment guidelines. An understanding of absolute and relative risk is essential when making treatment decisions for individual patients.

> Treatment decisions should be based on a formal estimation of 10-year coronary heart disease risk using the programme 'Cardiac Risk Assessor' or the coronary heart disease risk chart issued by the Joint British Societies. The treatment threshold is flexible, based on the level of blood pressure and the total cardiovascular risk. For example, a blood pressure of 140/85 mmHg is normal in a low-risk individual, but should be treated in a diabetic with a high overall cardiovascular risk.

Cardiovascular risk estimation according to age: the risk of under-treating the young and over-treating the elderly

All patients should have a global or total cardiovascular risk estimation based on their risk profile, organ damage and disease. The risk should be categorised as low, moderate, high or very high. The estimated risk determines the treatment strategy, whether the patient should be treated, the target blood pressure level, the use of combination therapies, and the need for a statin and other non-hypertensive drugs.

The commonly used British Societies' risk tables are based on Framingham data, which apply to only some European and US populations. The SCORE model is recommended by the European Society of Cardiology, available on their website (www.escardio.org).

An understanding of absolute and relative risk is important when deciding upon treatment for patients with hypertension. An individual's cardiovascular risk is recorded using risk charts to estimate their *absolute risk* of a cardiovascular event over the next 10 years. Risk estimation is used to make treatment decisions 'intelligent' so that limited resources are targeted to those most at risk. In the UK, the guidelines recommend treatment only if an individual's risk of a cardiovascular event over the next 10 years is greater than 20%. This is an arbitrary cut-off value and is not universally used. Risk estimates are inaccurate, and strict adherence to this treatment threshold would mean that an individual who was estimated to be at a marginally lower risk would not be treated.

Age is a heavily weighted risk factor. An elderly patient's *absolute risk* is much higher than that of a young patient, almost irrespective of their level of blood pressure and the presence of other risk factors. Most men aged over 70 years will justify treatment, although their relative risk will be similar to that of their 'normal' peers. The absolute risk in a young woman is unlikely to reach treatment thresholds, even if she has a major risk factor, although she is at much higher relative risk compared with a woman of the same age without risk factors.

The consequence of basing treatment on absolute rather than relative risk is that most resources would be concentrated on older people, whose long-term mortality may not be improved, although their cardiovascular event rate may be reduced. Less attention is paid to preventing cardiovascular disease in young people who may be at significant long-term risk and who may develop irreversible cardiovascular problems when still relatively young. To reduce long-term risk in young patients, treatment deci-sions should be guided by their *relative risk* (their risk compared with that of people of the same age who have no risk factors). These problems highlight the importance of using guidelines as guidelines and not as prescriptive protocols. Clinicians need to use evidence-based guidelines as a flexible foundation for deciding on treatment for each individual patient.

> In young patients, management should be based on relative rather than absolute risk.

Risk factors that influence prognosis in hypertension

These should be assessed and used to estimate risk in order to determine whether a patient should be treated. The decision to start treatment for hypertension depends on the blood pressure level and the patient's total cardiovascular risk. Levels above those given below constitute a significant risk factor.

The following risk factors influence prognosis in hypertension:

- levels of systolic and diastolic blood pressure
- pulse pressure in the elderly
- smoking
- dyslipidaemia:
    - total cholesterol >5.0 mmol/l or
    - LDL-cholesterol >3.0 mmol/l or
    - HDL-cholesterol <1.0 mmol/l
    - triglycerides >1.7 mmol/l
- fasting glucose 5.6–6.9 mmol/l
- abnormal glucose tolerance test
- family history of premature coronary artery disease (men aged <55 years and women aged <65 years)

- ✧ abdominal obesity (>102 cm in men and >88 cm in women)
- ✧ diabetes (fasting glucose >7.0 mmol/l, or random measurement >11.0 mmol/l)
- ✧ end-organ damage:
    - ∝ left ventricular hypertrophy on ECG or echocardiogram
    - ∝ carotid wall thickening or plaque
    - ∝ ankle-brachial blood pressure index <0.9
    - ∝ renal impairment (eGFR <60 ml/min)
    - ∝ microalbuminuria (30–300 mg/24 hours)
    - ∝ diabetes (fasting glucose >7.0 mmol/l)
- ✧ vascular disease in the brain, heart, kidneys, legs or eyes.

Metabolic syndrome

This is defined as the presence of three or more of the following: abdominal obesity, high fasting glucose, blood pressure >130/85 mmHg, low HDL-cholesterol levels and high triglyceride levels. It is most common in middle-aged and elderly patients, and is associated with a significantly higher cardiovascular risk. Other associated features include microalbuminuria, left ventricular hypertrophy and arterial stiffness.

Because patients are at greater risk, a more detailed investigation of sub-clinical organ damage is recommended. Twenty-four-hour ambulatory blood pressure recording and self-recorded blood pressure readings are helpful.

Angiotensin-converting-enzyme (ACE) inhibitors and/or angiotensin II receptor antagonists are recommended for treating hypertension in patients with metabolic syndrome. Calcium-channel blockers and/or thiazide diuretics can be added. β-blockers are not recommended as first-line therapy.

Statins and anti-diabetic medication are also used when necessary. The role of insulin sensitisers has not been defined.

Classification of cardiovascular risk

Classification of risk is easiest in individuals at high risk. It is most difficult and inaccurate in those who fall between high and low risk, and who are classified as intermediate risk.

High-risk individuals are those who have one or more of the following:

- ✧ systolic blood pressure >180 mmHg and/or diastolic pressure >110 mmHg
- ✧ any form of vascular disease
- ✧ metabolic syndrome
- ✧ organ damage (microalbuminuria – low-level albuminuria), left ventricular hypertrophy
- ✧ type 1 or type 2 diabetes mellitus
- ✧ one or more severely elevated risk factors
- ✧ older patients (men aged >55 years and women aged >65 years).

Low-risk individuals are those who:

- ✧ are under 50 years of age
- ✧ have no risk factors.

Recording devices

Health and safety regulations have relegated the mercury sphygmomanometer to history in hospitals, which now use mainly automated, semi-automated and aneroid devices.

Measuring blood pressure

Blood pressure is a very labile haemodynamic parameter that varies with each heartbeat, hour of the day, season of the year, activity and position of the individual. Therefore, a diagnosis of hypertension should be based on many recordings made over several weeks. If blood pressure is only slightly high, many recordings should be taken over a period of months before a diagnosis of hypertension is made. However, if the patient has a very high recording and evidence of end-organ damage and other cardiovascular risk factors, the diagnosis is more secure.

> Blood pressure recordings can be taken not only by a doctor or nurse, but also by other trained healthcare professionals, and – assuming the recordings have been taken accurately under correct conditions – by the patient or carer at the patient's home.

Accurate recordings are inexpensive, easily obtained, non-invasive determinants of cardiovascular status and cardiovascular events.

⋄ Blood pressure should be measured with the patient sitting at ease and as relaxed as possible, in a quiet room (or standing if elderly or diabetic, or if orthostatic hypertension is suspected). Two recordings separated by at least one minute should be taken, and more if the recordings are very different. Measure the blood pressure in both arms at the first visit, to investigate the possibility of coarctation. The patient should be relaxed.

⋄ Current guidelines recommend that recordings should be taken in all patients at least every five years, but the frequency of recordings will be determined by the patient's clinical state. Patients with borderline readings and those with hypertension that is difficult to control will require more frequent recordings and clinical assessments.

⋄ The recording device should be validated, calibrated and regularly maintained. The blood pressure cuff must be of an appropriate size for the patient's arm, which should be at the level of the heart, and the cuff must be deflated slowly enough to aim to measure the blood pressure to the nearest 2 mmHg.

⋄ The cuff should be inflated above the systolic level by feeling the brachial artery pulsation disappear as the cuff is inflated. The stethoscope should then be applied over the brachial artery as the cuff is gradually and slowly deflated.

⋄ The systolic pressure should be recorded as the level when the pulse sounds reappear with cuff deflation (Korotkov phase 1). The diastolic level should be recorded as the pulse sounds disappear (Korotkov phase 5). The average of at least two readings should be taken.

✧ Because of the weighting given to blood pressure in cardiovascular risk assessment, use the average recording from several visits when estimating the 10-year risk.

White-coat syndrome

In white coat syndrome, the blood pressure in the surgery is >140/90 mmHg, but the home recording is <130/85 mmHg. Cardiovascular risk is less than in individuals with raised surgery and ambulatory or home recordings.

Self-measurement of blood pressure

Self-measurement of blood pressure is of clinical and prognostic value. The normal value of home, self-recorded blood pressure is <130–135/85 mmHg. Doctors used to be reluctant to advise patients to record their own blood pressure, because they were not confident about the accuracy of the recordings, which may be taken when patients are stressed or anxious, or shortly after exercising. However, in the same way as some people like to check their weight, or measure their heart rate while exercising (both of which are sensible things to do), self-recording devices are popular with some patients who like to keep an eye on their blood pressure to check whether they are 'healthy' and their blood pressure is within normal limits. Accurate recordings assist the evaluation of treatment, and encourage patients to take their tablets.

However, some patients may become obsessed with their blood-pressure measurements, and this is undesirable. If patients become obsessed and feel anxious, they should be advised to stop taking their blood pressure. Patients should be told that irrespective of their recordings, they must not alter their medication without consulting their doctor.

There are several blood-pressure machines available for self-recording. In general, semi-automatic arm recorders are more accurate than wrist recorders. The patient should sit while measuring their blood pressure, and should have rested for several minutes beforehand. Recordings should not be taken shortly after exercise or if the patient feels stressed. Self-recorded home measurements are lower than clinic or surgery recordings. It is useful for patients to check their device and the accuracy of their self-recording against a simultaneous recording performed in the surgery.

Ambulatory blood-pressure recording

This is a very useful and accurate method for non-invasive measurement of the blood pressure during usual daily activities over a 24-hour period. It provides blood-pressure data when the patient is asleep, driving, working or engaged in activities that would be expected to have a significant effect on blood pressure, and when self-recordings or clinic recordings would be difficult to obtain. Many GP surgeries now have their own machines as well as software on their computers to analyse the data, and this greatly improves the quality of care for patients with established or suspected hypertension.

Ambulatory blood pressure recordings are much stronger predictor of cardiovascular morbidity and mortality than conventional blood-pressure recordings. Ambulatory blood-pressure recording should be available to all patients with known or suspected hypertension.

Ambulatory blood-pressure recordings have shown the natural circadian variation in blood pressure, with an early-morning surge, which accounts for the peak incidence of cardiac and cerebrovascular events in the morning. High recordings are associated with stress, and low levels are recorded when the patient is asleep or resting. This type of recording provides a full 24-hour 'panorama' of the patient's blood pressure, rather than a 'snapshot' measurement taken when both the patient and possibly the GP or nurse are stressed in a busy clinic.

Ambulatory blood-pressure recordings and white-coat syndrome (hypertension only in clinic or the surgery)

Twenty-four-hour ambulatory blood pressure recording is particularly helpful for evaluating the possibility of white-coat syndrome, which is present in around 15% of the general population.

> White-coat hypertension is defined as high clinic readings (>140/90 mmHg) but normal ambulatory blood pressure recordings (<130/80 mmHg), apart from the first stressful and unfamiliar hour of the ambulatory recording.

Although patients with this common condition do not generally appear to benefit from antihypertensive treatment, the prevalence of end-organ damage is higher than in individuals without white-coat syndrome, so it is not a completely benign condition. Patients with white-coat syndrome should be screened for risk factors and organ damage.

> Antihypertensive medication is recommended for patients with white-coat syndrome who have cardiovascular risk factors or organ damage.

Patients who have raised clinic recordings but an average 24-hour blood pressure level of <130/80 mmHg are no more likely than normotensive people to have a cardiovascular event. They do not need medication unless they have significant risk factors or organ damage, and thus drug side effects are avoided. Excluding hypertension has important employment and insurance benefits for the patient and reduces healthcare costs.

Ambulatory blood-pressure recordings are a better predictor of cardiovascular outcomes than isolated clinic recordings in patients with treated hypertension. High ambulatory recordings (a mean blood pressure of >135/85 mmHg), particularly at night, are also reliable in predicting cardiovascular events. Patients with raised clinic blood pressure recordings should be considered for ambulatory recordings.

Indications for 24-hour ambulatory blood-pressure recording
- Diagnosis of white-coat syndrome.
- Deciding the diagnosis in patients with borderline clinic readings.
- Marked variability of clinic recordings.

✧   Resistant hypertension (>150/90 mmHg despite three or more drugs).
✧   Suspected hypotension, particularly in diabetics or the elderly.
✧   Patients with a blood pressure of >160/100 mmHg with no target organ damage and an estimated 10-year cardiovascular risk of <15%. If the average ambulatory blood pressure recording is normal, medication may not be necessary.
✧   Deciding on treatment in elderly patients with isolated systolic hypertension.
✧   Patients with hypertension in pregnancy.
✧   When a previous ambulatory blood pressure recording is normal but the patient has borderline hypertension or significant cardiovascular risk for other reasons.
✧   Evaluation of the efficacy of treatment.
✧   Sleep apnoea.

Interpreting the results of ambulatory blood-pressure recording

Patients should be asked to fill in a diary recording their activities during the day, when they rested and went to bed, and how well they slept. They should not exercise vigorously while wearing the cuff. They can take the cuff off when they have a bath or shower. At least 70% of the recordings should be 'valid' and not affected by artefact.

The decision to treat should be based on the average daytime readings, not the average 24-hour recording. The threshold for starting treatment should be 12/7 mmHg lower than clinic readings, because blood pressure recordings are systematically lower with ambulatory recordings. Thus, an average ambulatory recording of 148/83 mmHg, which equates to a clinic blood pressure of 160/90 mmHg, may require treatment.

> An average ambulatory blood pressure of 130/80 mmHg is normal in low-risk individuals, but a level of <120/75 mmHg is optimal in diabetics.

Ambulatory 24-hour blood-pressure recordings identify patients whose blood pressure does not fall normally at night – so-called 'non-dippers' – who are probably at high risk.

Exercise-induced hypertension

Blood pressure increases with both mental stress and physical exercise.

High blood-pressure values resulting from mental stress have been found to predict those who develop hypertension later in life.

Normally, during exercise, the systolic blood pressure increases and the diastolic pressure falls. These changes rely on an intact response of the peripheral vessels (reduced systemic vascular resistance to leg exercise), a normal heart pump and blood supply, and a normal autonomic nervous system. An exaggerated blood-pressure response to exercise (peak exercise-related systolic blood pressure >200 mmHg) may identify patients with hypertension who have not been previously diagnosed. It also predicts cardiovascular death, and therefore adds prognostic information.

Causes of hypertension

> The most common cause of hypertension is 'essential hypertension', which accounts for at least 94% of cases.

Secondary causes of hypertension
Renal parenchymal disease

Renal parenchymal disease is the most common cause of secondary hypertension. It is suggested by urinalysis that shows erythrocytes, white cells and protein. Referral and further investigations are warranted. Two normal creatinine levels and urinalyses exclude renal parenchymal disease.

> Urinalysis and creatinine levels should be measured in all patients with hypertension to investigate the presence of renal parenchymal disease.

Bilateral polycystic kidney disease may be found on clinical examination. Ultrasound is diagnostic.

Hypertension may result from acute renal failure of any cause, including acute glomerulonephritis, vasculitis, acute obstruction, or chronic renal failure due to diabetic nephropathy or chronic glomerulonephritis.

Management

The threshold for treatment in patients with renal disease is >140/90 mmHg, and the target is <130/85 mmHg. These patients should be referred to a specialist to plan and monitor the long-term management of the underlying renal disease and to choose the most appropriate combination of tablets. Thiazide diuretics (e.g. bendroflumethiazide, indapamide, hydrochlorothiazide) may be ineffective and high-dose loop diuretics (furosemide) may be required. Aggressive lowering of the blood pressure may slow progression of the renal disease. Salt restriction is important in patients with impaired renal function. Patients should be considered for aspirin and statins.

Renovascular hypertension

This is the second-most common cause of secondary hypertension, accounting for 2% of hypertensive patients referred to specialist centres. Reduced blood flow to either or both kidneys, due to renal artery stenosis, results in activation of the renin–angiotensin system, with increased renin levels and fluid retention. There are two causes of renal artery stenosis.

❖ *Atherosclerotic disease* (70% of cases) usually affects both renal arteries (although it is often more marked in one artery), and is a progressive disease. It should be considered in patients with resistant hypertension and those who have evidence or a high probability of vascular disease, those who have smoked, those with peripheral vascular, cerebrovascular or coronary artery disease, and those who develop increasing renal impairment when treated with ACE inhibitors or angiotensin II antagonists. Bilateral renal artery stenosis may cause 'flash pulmonary oedema' with normal left ventricular failure.

✧ *Fibromuscular dysplasia* (25% of cases) occurs typically in young females who present with hypertension and no family history of hypertension.

Diagnosis and management

Patients with suspected renal artery stenosis should be referred for a specialist opinion. Features include an abdominal bruit, hypokalaemia and progressive decline in renal function. Colour flow Doppler ultrasound, computerised tomography (CT) and magnetic resonance scanning can be used to select patients for arteriography and revascularisation with angioplasty and stenting (which can be performed at the same time as arteriography), or surgical reconstruction of the affected arteries. Three-dimensional, gadolinium-enhanced, magnetic resonance angiography may prove to be the diagnostic procedure with the highest accuracy.

Fibromuscular renal artery stenosis

Angioplasty and stenting are useful in patients with fibromuscular renal artery stenosis.

Renal angioplasty may be complicated by local problems. These include proteinuria following a sudden increase in renal artery pressure after dilatation of the stenosis, radiographic contrast-agent-induced renal damage, cholesterol emboli (in atherosclerotic disease) and restenosis in 50% of patients.

Atherosclerotic renal artery stenosis

Renal angioplasty is no more effective for control of blood pressure than antihypertensive drug therapy alone in atherosclerotic renal artery stenosis. It is therefore no longer necessary to screen all hypertensive patients for renal artery stenosis with a view to angioplasty. However, it should be considered for those with uncontrolled hypertension, high serum creatinine levels, bilateral renal artery stenosis (which may present as 'flash pulmonary oedema') and severe unilateral renal artery stenosis.

All classes of antihypertensive drugs may be used. ACE inhibitors may be used in uni-lateral renal artery stenosis, but are contraindicated in severe bilateral disease. All patients on ACE inhibitors need regular renal function tests. Increases in serum creatinine levels are usually reversed when the ACE inhibitor is stopped. In patients who are on maximal medical treatment but who have resistant severe hypertension, the risk of continuing ACE inhibitors must be weighed against the dangers of uncontrolled hypertension. These patients require specialist assessment.

Aortic coarctation

This is a narrowing of the aorta, usually distal to the left subclavian artery, and may be associated with a bicuspid aortic valve and other heart defects. It should be diagnosed in childhood. Affected patients may have a systolic heart murmur heard over the chest and back, hypertension and decreased leg pulses. The blood pressure is high in the arms but often unrecordable in the legs and feet. The resulting hypertension usually resolves if the coarctation is resected during childhood. Stenting can also be used. Hypertension usually persists if surgery is performed in a patient over 40 years of age. Affected patients are vulnerable to hypertensive complications at a younger age.

Management

These patients should be referred for investigation and consideration of surgery or angioplasty. Even after correction of the coarctation, patients require follow-up for hypertension and its complications.

Cushing's syndrome

Hypertension affects 80% of patients with Cushing's syndrome, thus accounting for less than 0.1% of the total population. The diagnosis can be made on the basis of the typical physical appearance.

Management

A 24-hour urinary cortisol level of >110 mmol/l suggests the diagnosis. This is confirmed with a two-day low-dose dexamethasone suppression test (0.5 mg every six hours for eight doses). In the two-day test a urinary cortisone excretion rate higher than 27 mmol/l per day on day two is diagnostic of Cushing's syndrome. A normal result excludes the diagnosis. Patients should be referred for investigation and management of the underlying problem, but also require effective treatment for hypertension.

Conn's syndrome (primary hyperaldosteronism)

This condition is most commonly due to a benign, unilateral, autonomous adenoma of the adrenal gland secreting aldosterone. This results in low renin levels, increased sodium levels and low potassium levels, particularly in patients who are taking diuretics. Importantly, most patients have normal plasma electrolytes at presentation. Conn's syndrome accounts for 1% of patients with hypertension. Around 70% of cases are due to adrenal hyperplasia.

Around 30% of cases are due to adrenal adenomas, which are more common in women. The condition should be suspected in people with hypokalaemia and in those with resistant hypertension.

Management

These patients should be referred for confirmation and categorisation of the diagnosis and guidance on the most appropriate medical treatment, which is often necessary. Diagnosis is made by measuring 24-hour urinary aldosterone. The plasma aldosterone : plasma renin ratio after withdrawing antihypertensive treatment for two weeks is used, but interpretation of this test is difficult and controversial. Primary aldosteronism can be confirmed by the fludrocortisone suppression test (failure of four-day administration of the hormone to reduce plasma aldosterone and renin levels).

Aldosterone-secreting adenomata should be localised by either CT or MRI scanning. Adrenal hyperplasia may produce false-positive scan results. Adenomas should be removed because this leads to resolution of hypertension in 70% of cases.

Phaeochromocytoma

These catecholamine-secreting tumours are usually unilateral and limited to the adrenal glands. They account for 0.2% of cases of hypertension. They may present incidentally as a first hypertensive episode peri-operatively, or as episodic hypertension, headache, and palpitation with or without tachycardia, pallor and sweating. Other symptoms reflecting catecholamine excess include anxiety, tremor, nausea, chest or abdominal pain, weight loss and fatigue. There may be dramatic elevations in blood pressure.

The diagnosis should be suspected in patients with suggestive symptoms, resistant hypertension or severe hypertension during pregnancy, when the uterus may press on the adrenal gland.

Management

The diagnosis can be made by measuring the levels of catecholamines in the blood, or catecholamine breakdown products in the urine over a 24-hour collection period. The most sensitive test (98%) is the level of plasma-free metanephrines, but this is not widely available. The 24-hour urinary catecholamine level is the most commonly performed test. If the level is very high, no further diagnostic tests are required. Localisation of the tumour is then necessary. Around 95% of these tumours are located close to or in the adrenal glands. Large ones can be seen on ultrasound. CT is more sensitive (>98%). A negative assay has a 98% predictive value for excluding the condition in a primary care population, and the test may be arranged with the local pathology department, which will be able to provide instructions on what the patient should do about food and medication before and during the collection.

Patients should be referred to a specialist who may wish to perform further tests, including localisation of the tumour by MRI or CT scanning. Surgical removal of the tumour(s) (now performed laparoscopically) usually results in normalisation of the blood pressure, but 25% of patients may have persistent hypertension.

Sleep apnoea

Patients with this condition are usually very overweight and stop breathing for periods while asleep. Sleep apnoea can be very worrying for the patient's partner. It can cause blood pressure that is resistant to treatment in obese individuals. Patients feel sleepy during the day and find it difficult to concentrate, and choke while asleep. Sleep studies using polysomnography are used to diagnose the condition. The problem usually responds to substantial weight loss and the use of positive pressure breathing equipment at night.

Drug causes of hypertension

All prescribed and non-prescribed medication should be noted. The following drugs cause hypertension:

◇ oestrogens and oral contraceptives
◇ β-agonists (bronchodilators, stimulant abuse, over-the-counter 'cold cures')
◇ steroids
◇ liquorice
◇ non-steroidal anti-inflammatory drugs
◇ amphetamines.

Contributory and correctable factors in relation to hypertension

◇ Being overweight.
◇ Excess alcohol consumption (>three units per day).
◇ Excess salt intake.
◇ Lack of exercise.

Complications and target organ damage

◇ Stroke and/or transient ischaemic attack.
◇ Multi-infarct dementia.
◇ Left ventricular hypertrophy.
◇ Heart failure.
◇ Coronary artery disease.
◇ Peripheral arterial disease.
◇ Retinal hypertensive changes.
◇ Proteinuria.
◇ Renal impairment (raised serum creatinine, microalbuminuria).

Rationale for effective treatment of hypertension

Hypertension increases the risk of vascular diseases, particularly stroke and coronary heart disease and renal disease.

Reducing cardiovascular risk necessitates treatment of hypertension and all other risk factors. Blood pressure values in the range 130–139/85–89 mmHg are associated with a greater than two-fold increase in the relative risk of cardiovascular disease compared with the risk for people with a blood pressure of 120/80 mmHg. Reducing blood pressure by 12/6 mmHg reduces the risk of stroke by 40% and that of coronary disease by 20%.

Those at highest cardiovascular risk derive the most benefit from treatment of hypertension.

Lowering blood pressure reduces fatal and non-fatal cardiovascular events. Treatment of hypertension in the elderly reduces the risk of dementia. Treatment of hypertension in people aged over 80 years reduces the risk of stroke and myocardial infarction.

All classes of antihypertensive drugs appear to be similar in their effects.

Aims and principles of treatment

- The aim is to achieve maximal reduction in the long-term risk of cardiovascular disease.
- Treatment should start before end-organ damage and cardiovascular disease occur.
- The blood pressure should be reduced to target levels, and all associated reversible risk factors should be treated.
- Blood pressure should be reduced to below 140/90 mmHg, and to lower levels if tolerated, in all patients.
- In diabetics, patients with renal impairment and proteinuria, and those with vascular disease (stroke, myocardial infarction), the target level is <130/80 mmHg.
- Patients aged over 80 years should be treated in a similar way to patients aged over 55 years.
- Isolated systolic hypertension (systolic blood pressure >160 mmHg) should be treated in the same way as combined systolic and diastolic hypertension.
- Most patients will need more than one antihypertensive drug to achieve target levels.
- Compliance is better if once-daily dosing is used.
- Non-proprietary drugs reduce treatment costs.
- Patients should be advised about common side effects so that they can make informed choices about their treatment.
- Treatment should be started if the blood pressure is >160/100 mmHg, and if it is >140/85 mmHg in patients with vascular disease and those with an estimated 10-year cardiovascular risk of >20%.
- Patients with accelerated (malignant) hypertension (papilloedema, fundal haemorrhages or exudates) should be referred and admitted to hospital for immediate treatment, but treatment should be started in the surgery if there is a delay in hospital admission.
- Treatment should be started immediately in patients with a blood pressure of >220/120 mmHg.
- Drug therapy should be started in all patients with sustained (monitored over a four-week period) systolic blood pressure of >160 mmHg or sustained diastolic blood pressure of >100 mmHg despite non-pharmacological measures.
- Drug therapy should be started in patients with sustained systolic blood pressure >140 mmHg or diastolic blood pressure >90 mmHg *only* if:
  - target organ damage is present, *or*
  - there is evidence of cardiovascular disease and/or diabetes, *or*
  - the 10-year coronary heart disease risk is >15%.

Otherwise, patients with a blood pressure of <160/100 mmHg and *no* target organ damage or cardiovascular complications, no diabetes and a 10-year coronary heart disease risk of <15% do not need drug treatment, but should be given advice about non-pharmacological measures and be monitored monthly.

✧ Patients with a blood pressure of <135/85 mmHg should be reassessed every five years.

The aim of treatment is to lower blood pressure sufficiently to prevent cardiovascular complications with no drug-induced adverse effects. The choice of drug is of secondary importance.

Response to treatment is mainly determined by the patient's age, assuming that there is good compliance.

Patient education

One of the major problems in treating hypertension is that most patients are symptom-free and do not like taking tablets. Treatment means total management, not just tablets. It is important that patients understand what hypertension is, what their blood pressure is and what their target level is, what the risks of uncontrolled hypertension are, what general measures they can and should instigate and maintain for themselves to reduce blood pressure and cardiovascular risk, what tablets they should take, and how frequently they should be monitored. They should understand that treatment is for life and that when their blood pressure becomes controlled they must continue to take tablets, and these may need to be increased if their blood pressure increases.

Although the prevention of cardiovascular complications is the principal aim and, hopefully, result of treatment, antihypertensive treatment also prevents dementia, which suggests that it improves the quality of life both mentally and physically in symptom-free patients.

After establishing a diagnosis of hypertension, patients need to understand that treatment and lifestyle measures are for life. Medication may need to be adjusted or changed depending on the response or the development of side effects.

Blood pressure targets

Targets are helpful to clinicians, but are difficult to achieve even in fully compliant patients. The blood pressure levels suggested as 'audit standards' in the current guidelines are higher than the recommended targets. These different levels cause confusion.

Because blood pressure increases with age, life events and other factors, the recommended targets become increasingly difficult to achieve. Blood pressure reduction, particularly reduction of systolic pressure in people aged over 60 years, is important in reducing cardiovascular events.

> In general, the lower the blood pressure the better, particularly in diabetics.
> The target for all patients of all ages is <140/90 mmHg.
> The target for patients with diabetes and/or target organ damage or cardio-vascular disease is <130/80 mmHg.

When the target blood pressure is not achieved

Patients with resistant hypertension may become anxious and feel that they have 'failed' by not achieving their blood-pressure target. They should be told that resistant hypertension is not uncommon even with perfect compliance and appropriate medication. Occasionally, this anxiety and frustration may lead to a preoccupation with their blood-pressure levels, making control more difficult. When starting drug therapy, it may be helpful to advise patients that it may not be possible to achieve the target blood pressure despite perfect compliance and the best medication. Further emphasis on non-pharmacological measures is often helpful to the patient's morale.

Target achievers

Some responders may feel that the diagnosis was wrong and may stop or ask to stop their tablets. If hypertensive patients stop taking their tablets, their blood pressure will inevitably increase within a few weeks, but it may occasionally be necessary to go through this exercise in order to convince doubtful patients.

TABLE 4.3 Target blood pressures during antihypertensive treatment (both the systolic and diastolic blood pressure targets should be attained)

	CLINIC BLOOD PRESSURE (MMHG)		MEAN DAYTIME ABPM OR HOME BLOOD PRESSURE (MMHG)	
	No diabetes	Diabetes	No diabetes	Diabetes
Optimal BP	<140/85	<130/80	<130/80	<130/75
Audit standard[a]	<150/90	<140/85	<140/85	<140/80

ABPM, ambulatory blood pressure monitoring.

a The audit standard is the minimum recommended level of blood pressure control, recognising that only 10% of patients have blood levels at target.

Target achievers should be congratulated on achieving their targets and reassured that the reason why their blood pressure is 'low' is because of the medication and other measures they are taking.

Non-pharmacological measures

Quite often, overweight, stressed, inactive people with high clinic blood pressure readings respond to the measures listed below, which are effective and may make drug treatment unnecessary, or at least reduce the number of different drugs needed by enhancing the antihypertensive effect of the drugs. These measures are effective, safe and – compared with drug treatment – inexpensive. Patients need enthusiastic supervision, monitoring, encouragement, and regular supervision and support. These measures are an integral part of the initial and long-term treatment of all patients with hypertension. Drug treatment may need to be started without delay in patients with severe hypertension.

There is no evidence from controlled trials that complementary therapies (e.g. foods, acupuncture, hypnosis, spinal manipulation, herbal therapies) are as effective as conventional drug therapies.

The following non-pharmacological methods are effective:

✧ weight loss to achieve optimal weight and body shape
✧ reduction of salt intake to less than 5 g (1 teaspoonful) per day
✧ low-fat diet
✧ modest alcohol consumption (<7 units per week for men and women). There is no controlled trial evidence on what is a 'safe' level of alcohol consumption. High levels of alcohol consumption lead to obesity and hypertension. The mode of action of alcohol on blood pressure is unclear
✧ cardiovascular exercise (e.g. 30 minutes of fast walking per day and avoidance of heavy isometric exercise)
✧ a diet rich in fruit and vegetables, rather than one with a high fat, salt and sugar content (as found in processed and 'ready meals')
✧ stopping smoking
✧ optimisation of lipids with drugs if necessary.

Treatment thresholds

These are based on an estimation of coronary heart disease risk.

> Effective antihypertensive treatment results in a relative risk reduction of 38% for stroke and 16% for coronary events.

The pros and cons of drug treatment have to be explained to patients who reach the treatment thresholds. Ultimately it is the responsibility of the patient to comply with the advice given, but additional consultations are helpful in addressing concerns that they or their family may have.

Choice of antihypertensive drug

The British Hypertension Society has provided useful information on indications and contraindications for different classes of antihypertensive drugs (*see* Table 4.4).

TABLE 4.4 Indications and contraindications of antihypertensive drugs

CLASS OF DRUG	INDICATIONS	CONTRAINDICATIONS
ACE inhibitors	Heart failure	Pregnancy
	Left ventricular dysfunction	Renovascular disease
	Diabetic nephropathy	PVD[b]
	Chronic renal disease[a]	Hyperkalaemia
	Previous MI	
	Metabolic syndrome	
	Diabetes	
β-blockers[c]	Myocardial infarction	Asthma/COAD
	Angina	Heart block
	Heart failure[d]	Bradycardia
	Women of childbearing age	Severe claudication
	Intolerance to ACE/ARB	Metabolic syndrome
	Atrial fibrillation	Diabetes
	Glaucoma	Athletes and physically active
Calcium-channel blockers (dihydropyridines)	Elderly ISH	
	Angina	
	Inadequate control with β-blockers	
	Claudication	
	Afro-Caribbeans	
Calcium-channel blockers (rate-limiting)	Angina	Heart block
	Uncontrolled atrial fibrillation	Bradycardia
		Heart failure
Thiazides	Elderly	Gout
		Glucose intolerance
		Pregnancy
α-blockers	Prostatism	Postural hypotension
	Dyslipidaemias	Urinary incontinence
Antialdosterone diuretic		Renal failure
		Hyperkalaemia

ISH, isolated systolic hypertension; ACE inhibitor, angiotensin-converting-enzyme inhibitor; ARB, angiotensin-receptor blocker; MI, myocardial infarction.

a ACE inhibitors may be beneficial in chronic renal failure, but should be used with caution, with monitoring of renal function and specialist advice if the patient has severe renal impairment.

b PVD (peripheral vascular disease) is a possible contraindication to ACE inhibitors because of its association with renal artery stenosis and renovascular disease.

c β-blockers can be continued in patients with well controlled hypertension if well tolerated, and should not be stopped in patients with angina or myocardial infarction.

d Use carefully (low dose to start with, and increasing slowly) in patients with significant left ventricular impairment or a history of heart failure.

Factors that influence the choice of antihypertensive drug

Table 4.4 provides useful clinical pointers when choosing an antihypertensive drug. The AB/CD rule is helpful when choosing drug combinations in hypertension, and refers to the first letter of the four main classes of drugs used.

Renin levels and hypertension

The recognition that younger (<55 years) Caucasian patients are more likely to have vasoconstrictor, high-renin hypertension (type 1), whereas Afro-Caribbean and older Caucasian patients tend to have volume-dependent, high-salt, low-renin hypertension (type 2), provides a pathophysiological rationale for choosing antihypertensive drugs.

- The high-renin, type 1 hypertensive patient should be treated with ACE inhibitors and/or angiotensin II antagonists (A) or β-blockers (B).
- Low-renin, type 2 hypertensive patients (e.g. Afro-Caribbean patients) have too much salt. They are best treated with a diuretic (D), or if they have resistant hypertension, with two different diuretics. A calcium antagonist (C) can be added, and they should have a low-salt diet. β-blockers and ACE inhibitors may be ineffective as monotherapy, although these drugs may be used when combined with a drug that activates the renin–angiotensin system (e.g. diuretics, calcium antagonists or α-blockers).
- For both types of hypertension, dietary measures are important. Compared with patients who have type 2 hypertension, salt restriction in patients with type 1 hypertension may not be as effective in reducing blood pressure.

Drug combinations

Drugs from different classes have additive effects when combined. Sub-maximal doses of two drugs may avoid or reduce side effects from maximal doses of a single drug. The A or B + C or D rule applies.

Rational drug combinations are as follows:

- a diuretic (D) + either a β-blocker (B) or an ACE inhibitor or angiotensin II antagonist (A), *or*
- a calcium antagonist (C) + either a β-blocker (B) or an ACE inhibitor or angiotensin II antagonist (A)
- if a third antihypertensive drug is necessary, a calcium antagonist (C) can be added to a diuretic (D) and ACE inhibitor (A) and to a diuretic (D) and β-blocker (B).

Less than half of all hypertensives will be controlled on one drug, and one-third of patients will require three or more drugs.

Recommendations for treatment of hypertension

✧ In hypertensive patients over 55 years of age, or Afro-Caribbean patients of any age, the first choice for initial therapy should be either a calcium-channel blocker or a thiazide diuretic.

✧ In hypertensive patients under 55 years of age, the first choice for initial therapy should be an ACE inhibitor or an angiotensin-II receptor antagonist if the ACE inhibitor is not tolerated.

✧ If initial therapy was with a calcium-channel blocker or a thiazide diuretic, and a second drug is required, add an ACE inhibitor. If initial therapy was with an ACE inhibitor, add a calcium-channel blocker or a thiazide-type diuretic.

✧ If treatment with three drugs is required, the combination of an ACE inhibitor, a calcium-channel blocker and a thiazide diuretic should be used.

✧ If the blood pressure is still not controlled on three drugs, add a fourth drug (another diuretic, an α-blocker or a β-blocker). Careful monitoring of renal function is necessary if two diuretics are used.

✧ When blood pressure is not controlled, consider non-compliance. A specialist opinion may be required.

✧ β-blockers are no longer recommended for *initial* treatment of hypertension. They are used in young patients who cannot tolerate ACE inhibitors or angiotensin-II receptor antagonists, and in women of child-bearing age. In these circumstances, a calcium-channel blocker should be added to the β-blocker.

✧ β-blockers do *not* need to be stopped in patients whose blood pressure is well controlled (<140/90 mmHg).

✧ β-blockers should be continued in patients for whom there are compelling reasons for β-blockade (angina or myocardial infarction), unless there are significant side effects.

✧ β-blocker doses should be reduced gradually.

✧ An ACE inhibitor would be appropriate for patients with diabetes and/or vascular disease.

✧ For patients with cardiac failure, a combination of a diuretic and an ACE inhibitor plus a β-blocker is appropriate.

✧ Dihydropyridine calcium antagonists can be used as an alternative to a diuretic in elderly patients with isolated systolic hypertension, and these have been shown to prevent strokes.

✧ Drug treatment is generally for life.

Monitoring response to treatment

Follow-up is essential to assess the patient's response to treatment. The aim of treatment is to achieve the target blood pressure without intolerable side effects. Some patients may need to be reviewed every few weeks initially. Six-monthly review is recommended for patients with well-controlled hypertension and no organ damage or renal impairment. Home recordings allow less frequent surgery review.

Follow-up allows the clinician to review all of the cardiovascular risk factors.

It may be possible to reduce antihypertensive medication in patients who were previously overweight and taking little exercise, but who have now become slim and fit.

Inappropriate drug combinations

The following drug combinations are not recommended:

✧ β-blocker + verapamil or diltiazem (bradycardia)
✧ ACE inhibitor + angiotensin II antagonist (renal failure and hyperkalaemia)
✧ potassium-sparing diuretic + ACE inhibitor.

Compliance

> Drugs don't work if they are not taken.
>   Is treatment failure due to the drug or to the patient?

However appropriate and rational the choice of antihypertensive drugs, there is little chance of lowering the patient's blood pressure if they do not take their medication as prescribed. It is essential that patients understand why, despite feeling well, they need to take tablets as prescribed for life, and that medications may need to be increased if their blood pressure remains high.

Non-compliance is an important cause of failure to achieve blood-pressure targets. Failure to recognise this leads to the clinician prescribing a higher dose of the prescribed medication or alternative additional tablets. Most patients take approximately 75% of doses as prescribed across a variety of medical disorders. Compliance does not correlate with intelligence, personality, age, education or the number of drugs prescribed. Compliance is probably increased just before and after surgery appointments. Whether it is affected by whom the patient sees (GP or practice nurse) is unclear.

> Non-compliance should be suspected and explored as the first reason for persistent hypertension.

There are several reasons for non-compliance that may be viewed as 'part of human nature'.

✧ Non-compliance is more likely with frequent dosing during the day, and can be improved with once-daily dosing.
✧ Non-compliance may develop in previously compliant patients if they feel that the medication is not necessary or they become relaxed about their condition.
✧ Patients, particularly the elderly or those who are very busy, may simply forget to take the tablets at the prescribed times.

✧ Some patients may become lax and disinterested, perhaps because they feel that the medication is unnecessary.

Potential dangers of non-compliance

Patients may not take their tablets because they may be unconvinced that they need tablets for a condition that does not cause symptoms. Careful, and if necessary, repeated education is therefore important. Patients need to understand the risks of the condition and the benefits of treatment. The treatment side effects may be intolerable. Non-compliance is a common cause of resistant hypertension. Omission of short-acting drugs (e.g. calcium antagonists, β-blockers or vasodilators such as doxazocin) may result in blood-pressure surges with the risk of vascular events.

Improving drug compliance

Patient education is fundamental to compliance. The patient and their family must understand the risks of hypertension and the benefits to them of having their blood pressure controlled.

1. Select drugs that can be given together, preferably once a day and at a time that the patient will remember and schedule as part of their daily routine. Ask the patient what time of day they would prefer and would be more likely to remember their tablets. This depends on the patient having some routine to their day. This may be with their first cup of tea, with breakfast, on arriving at work or with lunch. Competent patients have to take responsibility for taking their medication. The patient's family can be helpful. Patients who travel frequently for work or social purposes need to establish a routine for taking their tablets.
2. Provide clear written information about the treatment and all non-pharmacological treatments.
3. Advise patients that self-recorded blood-pressure recordings may help them to take an interest in their condition.
4. Warn patients about possible important side effects, and advise them what to do if these occur. This is difficult because some patients attribute symptoms to the tablets. These problems can be dealt with at further reviews or by the practice nurse over the telephone.
5. Combination tablets, prescribed once a day, improve compliance.
6. Check compliance whenever the patient comes to the surgery.

Aspirin in hypertension

Treating a hypertensive patient with aspirin reduces cardiovascular events by 15% and myocardial infarction by 36%, but the benefit depends on the individual's absolute cardiovascular risk. The number of aspirin-related bleeds is similar to the number of cardiovascular events prevented by aspirin. Mortality is not affected. Therefore, aspirin confers only a marginal benefit.

Hypertension must be controlled before starting aspirin.

Aspirin is recommended in hypertension for primary prevention to patients:

✧ aged >50 years with target organ damage (left ventricular hypertrophy, proteinuria or renal impairment) with no contraindication *and* a blood pressure level of <150/90 mmHg

✧ with a 10-year coronary heart disease risk of >15% (antihypertensive treatment reduces this risk by 25%, and aspirin will reduce this risk by a further 15%)

✧ with type 2 diabetes.

The numbers needed to treat analysis for aspirin:

✧ 90 hypertensive patients will need to be treated with aspirin for five years in order to prevent one cardiovascular complication

✧ 60 hypertensive patients will need to be treated with aspirin for five years in order to prevent one myocardial infarct.

Aspirin is recommended in secondary prevention for patients with hypertension who have cardiovascular disease, provided that there is no excessive risk of bleeding.

Treating hypertension in diabetics

Hypertension is present in 70% of patients with type 2 diabetes, but its prevalence is not increased in patients with type 1 diabetes without nephropathy (microalbuminuria or proteinuria).

Insulin-treated diabetes without nephropathy

The threshold for drug intervention is >140/90 mmHg.

Insulin-treated diabetes with nephropathy

Blood pressure reduction and ACE inhibitors slow the rate of decline in renal function and delay progression to nephropathy.

Patients should be given an angiotensin II blocker if they cannot tolerate an ACE inhibitor. The blood pressure targets are 130/80 or 125/75 mmHg if there is proteinuria or albuminuria, respectively. Patients should be considered for aspirin and a statin.

ACE inhibitors are first-line treatment in diabetic patients, and should be given and titrated up to the maximum recommended and tolerated dose, even in patients who are normotensive.

Statins should be considered to achieve target levels of cholesterol <4.0 mmol/l and/or LDL <2.0 mmol/l.

Non-insulin-treated diabetes

Hypertension is common, related to obesity and predictive of cardiovascular events.

Weight loss to the patient's optimum weight and daily exercise are fundamental aspects of treatment.

Most diabetic patients will need two antihypertensive drugs.

> Hypertension control in diabetic patients is more important than glycaemic control in improving survival. It reduces the incidence of cardiovascular events by 50%.
> The recommended threshold for intervention with antihypertensive drugs in type 2 diabetes is <140/90 mmHg, and the target is <130/80 mmHg.

The choice of drugs, apart from using an ACE inhibitor, does not appear to matter.

Patients with type 2 diabetes and nephropathy are at high risk from cardiovascular events, and all of their risk factors need vigorous attention. They should have aspirin. The target blood pressure is 130/75 mmHg.

Treating hypertension in patients with kidney disease

Renal impairment is a major additional risk factor. Statins and aspirin are used with antihypertensive medication to reduce cardiovascular risk.

> The target blood pressure level is <130/80 mmHg.

Combination therapy is usually required.

An ACE inhibitor, with or without an angiotensin II receptor antagonist, is used to reduce proteinuria.

Lipid lowering in hypertension

Statins (with additional lipid-lowering drugs if necessary) are recommended to achieve a cholesterol concentration of <4.0 mmol/l and an LDL concentration of <2.0 mmol/l in:

✧ all hypertensive patients with cardiovascular disease and/or diabetes, *or*
✧ those whose 10-year cardiovascular risk is >20%.

Hypertension after myocardial infarction

β-blockers are recommended for all patients without contraindications after myocardial infarction, and ACE inhibitors for patients with left ventricular systolic impairment and for diabetic patients. All vascular risk factors should be treated.

Hypertension in women

Blood-pressure lowering is as beneficial in women as it is in men.

Oral contraceptives

All oral contraceptives, even those with a low oestrogen content, are associated with an increased risk of hypertension, stroke and myocardial infarction. The progestogen-only pill is an alternative option for women with hypertension, but there is little information on its influence on cardiovascular outcomes.

Hormone replacement therapy

The main indication for hormone replacement therapy (HRT) is for menopausal symptoms. HRT is not contraindicated in hypertensive women with severe flushing and other menopausal symptoms. It reduces the incidence of bone fractures and colon cancer, but is associated in certain high-risk groups with an increased risk of cardiovascular events, breast cancer, thromboembolism, gall-bladder disease and dementia. HRT is *not* recommended for cardiovascular protection in post-menopausal women.

Hypertension in pregnancy

Hypertension occurs in 10% of pregnancies, and is an important cause of maternal and fetal morbidity and mortality. It is associated with abruptio placentae and with cerebral haemorrhage in the mother, as well as fetal prematurity, stillbirth and neonatal death.

Hypertension may be the first sign of pre-eclampsia, which further increases the maternal and fetal risk and is characterised by significant proteinuria; oedema is no longer a diagnostic criterion. The mechanism of eclampsia remains unclear. It may lead to intrauterine growth restriction. The mother and the baby should be monitored carefully and may need referral to hospital if the blood pressure is not optimally controlled, if the baby is not growing or if there is proteinuria.

Hypertensive patients who become pregnant and those who develop hypertension during pregnancy should be referred to a cardiologist, who should liaise with obstetric colleagues to optimise management during pregnancy, delivery and postpartum.

Treatment thresholds during pregnancy

In the absence of evidence from randomised trials, treatment guidelines are based on observational studies, experience, and a reluctance to use drugs that could result in teratogenicity.

Blood-pressure levels fall during pregnancy, so it may be possible to reduce or withdraw medication in patients with mild hypertension, although frequent monitoring is essential.

Hospitalisation may be necessary, and drug treatment is essential in patients with a blood pressure of <170/110 mmHg. Drug treatment is also justified at levels of >140/90 mmHg. The blood pressure should be measured and the urine checked for protein every week. If either of these is unsatisfactory, the patient should be referred to hospital.

All women with hypertension during pregnancy should be monitored after delivery to ascertain whether they need long-term treatment or further investigations.

White-coat hypertension occurs in 30% of pregnant women. Ambulatory blood-pressure recordings are very useful, and the confirmation of a normal or only slightly raised blood pressure can avoid unnecessary anxiety, treatment and hospital admissions in this large group of individuals.

Pre-eclampsia

Patients are usually symptom-free, and 30% of pre-eclamptic fits occur in the absence of a raised blood pressure or proteinuria.

The diagnostic criteria are as follows:

- ✧ a rise in blood pressure of 15 mmHg diastolic or >30 mmHg systolic from early pregnancy, *or*
- ✧ a diastolic pressure of >90 mmHg on two occasions four hours apart or a diastolic pressure of >110 mmHg on one occasion and proteinuria.

Pre-eclampsia resolves with delivery, which has to be timed carefully to optimise fetal maturation.

Risk factors for pre-eclampsia include first pregnancy, change of partner, previous pre-eclampsia, family history of pre-eclampsia, idiopathic hypertension, chronic renal disease, diabetes, multiple pregnancy and obesity. Antihypertensive treatment has not been shown to improve fetal outcome.

> Patients with pre-eclampsia need urgent referral and treatment.

Choice of antihypertensive treatment in pregnancy

Methyldopa (750 mg to 4 g per day in three or four divided doses) remains the drug of choice because of its relatively low risk of side effects and the long experience of its use. Other acceptable drugs include calcium antagonists and labetolol. Diuretics reduce plasma volume and may theoretically increase the risk of pre-eclampsia. ACE inhibitors are contraindicated because of the risk of renal malformation.

Hypertensive women who become or plan to become pregnant should switch to a drug regime that is recommended as safe during pregnancy, and switch back to their usual medication after delivery.

Calcium supplementation, fish oil and low-dose aspirin are not recommended. Low-dose aspirin may be used prophylactically in women with a history of early-onset pre-eclampsia.

Resistant hypertension

This can be defined as a blood pressure above target levels despite treatment with three drugs in adequate dosage, after ensuring that the blood pressure has been correctly and accurately measured, and making sure that the patient is taking their tablets. This can be very difficult to confirm. Apart from white coat syndrome, it is important to consider lack of exercise, obesity, high-salt diet, excess alcohol consumption (the quantity depends on the patient, their age, gender and other unknown factors), taking of other drugs (cocaine, liquorice, glucocorticoids, non-steroidal anti-inflammatory drugs), obstructive sleep apnoea, unsuspected secondary causes of hypertension, and volume overload.

These patients should be referred for a specialist opinion and investigation.

Treatment of resistant hypertension

Compliance must first be checked, contributing factors addressed and secondary causes of hypertension, particularly phaeochromocytoma, hyperaldosteronism (Conn's syndrome) and renal artery stenosis, excluded. Patients with a high aldosterone : renin ratio may respond to spironolactone.

For patients who are already on four or five drugs, minoxidil, a powerful vasodilator, is effective. Its side effects include hirsutism (which may be welcomed in balding men).

A combination of a diuretic (D), a calcium antagonist (C), an ACE inhibitor (A) and/ or an α-blocker is usually effective.

Hypertension in the elderly

Isolated systolic hypertension is common in elderly patients but may be overestimated by clinic readings, leading to excessive treatment and possible side effects, including drug-related hypotension and falls. Thiazide diuretics, calcium antagonists and ACE inhibitors are useful and effective, and there is no clearly superior class of drug. Current guidelines recommend that renal function should be monitored if ACE inhibitors are used.

Ambulatory blood-pressure recordings are helpful when evaluating this group of patients. Management of the elderly hypertensive patient is no different to that for the younger patient. Dose increases should be gradual.

Emergency treatment of hypertension

This is indicated for:

◆ hypertensive encephalopathy (most often due to eclampsia)
◆ left ventricular failure
◆ dissecting aortic aneurysm
◆ hypertension with an acute coronary syndrome
◆ hypertension due to recreational drugs (cocaine, amphetamines, ecstasy)
◆ pre-eclampsia or eclampsia.

Intravenous nitrate alone or with labetolol is useful for lowering blood pressure in acute aortic dissection. Nitroprusside (for a maximum of a few days only, due to cyanide toxicity) can be used for the other two causes.

Advice for patients

✧ High blood pressure is common and becomes more common with age.

✧ Treatment is generally for life. If you stop taking your tablets, your blood pressure will probably increase after a few months. It is possible that your blood pressure may increase even though you take your tablets, and you may need a change in your treatment.

✧ There is a difference between feeling 'hyper' or anxious and having the medical condition of hypertension or high blood pressure. It is quite possible that people who are 'hyper' or anxious or stressed may have a high blood pressure at the time when they feel 'hyper'. However, this is normal and expected. Hypertension is a condition where the blood pressure is high all the time, and that is why we need to measure your blood pressure throughout the day.

✧ If the blood pressure in your arteries is high, they are subjected to strain and become stiff and liable to get furred up. This hardening of the arteries affects all of your arteries, and this is why people with a high blood pressure get complications.

✧ Even though you may not feel unwell, your blood pressure is too high, and this can lead to stroke, heart attack, a weakening of the heart, kidney damage, loss of sight and an unnecessarily early death. If we lower your blood pressure, your risk is lowered.

✧ Even though we are quite good at lowering blood pressure with tablets, we still do not know the cause of high blood pressure in nearly 95% of the people affected by it. However, we do know that high blood pressure is more common in people who are overweight, who don't exercise enough, who drink too much alcohol (more than two units per day) or who eat too much salt.

✧ If you smoke you should stop, because smoking increases your risk of having a serious heart problem or stroke.

✧ High blood pressure also runs in families, and there are some other unusual causes that account for around 5% of cases.

✧ If you want to check your own blood pressure, buy a good-quality machine that you put around your arm, and follow the instructions carefully. Bring it with you to the surgery and we will check its accuracy. If you feel anxious, it is possible that your pressure will be high. It may be that you do have high blood pressure, but we need to be sure that your high blood-pressure recordings are high enough for long enough to justify you taking blood-pressure tablets for the rest of your life.

✧ Your blood pressure will fall if you lose weight until you reach your 'best' weight and do regular exercise. If your blood pressure remains high despite this, then you will probably need tablets.

✧ The decision to give you tablets is complex, and is not based solely on your blood pressure recordings. We estimate your risk of developing heart disease on the basis of a number of factors – for example, your age, whether you have diabetes or a high cholesterol level, whether you have had a heart attack or whether you have furring up of your heart arteries.

✧ Because high blood pressure does not go away, if you have this condition you will need to take tablets for life, particularly as blood pressure increases in all of us as we get older. In general, the lower the blood pressure the better.

✧ Most people need to take at least two different types of tablets. The key point of treatment is to take enough tablets to lower the blood pressure to a safe level. If you think that you have a side effect to a tablet, come and see us and we will try to sort this out. There are several different tablets available, and we can usually find a combination that suits you, but we may not get the combination right at the first attempt!

✧ People with a low blood pressure live longer than those with a high pressure. A low blood pressure is not dangerous except if you feel faint when you stand up. The pressure needs to be lower than 90/60 mmHg before it results in you feeling light-headed. If you do feel like that, lie down quickly with your legs raised in the air. Come and see us and we will check this and see whether we need to adjust your tablets.

✧ People with controlled high blood pressure can and should lead a full and normal life. Driving, exercise and sports are to be encouraged.

✧ Holders of a passenger-carrying vehicle or large goods vehicle licence should inform the DVLA.

✧ Some men find that their sexual function deteriorates. If this happens, come to see us so that we can help. Sometimes it may be due to the tablets, but there are several causes that need to be investigated.

✧ Women who are on the oral contraceptive pill should have regular blood-pressure checks (at least every six months), because some formulations of the pill increase the blood pressure. The pill may need to be changed or stopped and another form of contraception used instead.

✧ Hypertensive women who are on HRT can continue with both treatments, but need to have their blood pressure checked.

✧ Women with high blood pressure who are pregnant need frequent blood pressure checks, and may need to have their tablets changed. In some women, the blood pressure is found to be high for the first time during pregnancy, and may remain high. Some women may need to be admitted to hospital for observation and treatment, or have their delivery induced before term.

Answers to questions about clinical cases

1. If a 24-hour blood pressure recording shows an average blood pressure of 135/85 mmHg or less, then the patient can be reassured and encouraged to exercise and lose weight. His blood sugar level will need review. If the 24-hour blood pressure recording is greater than 140/90 mmHg, he should be encouraged to pay serious attention to all of his risk factors and have another 24-hour blood pressure recording after he has lost weight and addressed all of the modifiable risk factors. If his blood pressure remains over 135/85 mmHg and a formal cardiovascular risk estimation indicates that he is at greater than 15% risk, he should be treated with either a thiazide or a β-blocker. Alternatively, if he is diagnosed as diabetic or cannot tolerate a β-blocker, he should be treated with an ACE inhibitor.

2. Treatment should be started immediately and the patient referred to hospital for further investigation.

3. If there is doubt about this patient's true daily blood-pressure recordings, check her 24-hour recordings. If these show a sustained rise in diastolic pressure of 15 mmHg, or a rise in systolic pressure of more than 30 mmHg, then she fulfils the criteria for pre-eclampsia and should be referred to hospital for treatment and control. Treatment should be started if the blood pressure is >170/110 mmHg, but many physicians would start treatment at a level of >140/90 mmHg. Even if the result of the 24-hour recording is satisfactory, this patient's blood pressure should be monitored continually during pregnancy and after delivery, because it is likely that she will require treatment at some stage.

4. Explain to the patient the potential advantages of blood-pressure control in reducing stroke, cardiovascular events, heart failure and dementia, and try her on a thiazide diuretic. Reducing her blood pressure is likely to prolong her active life. The target blood pressure level is 140/90 mmHg, and she may need an additional drug – for example, an ACE inhibitor.

5. Check the patient's blood pressure with an ambulatory recording. The target blood pressure for diabetics is <130/80 mmHg. At this level there is a 50% reduction in cardiovascular events. If her blood pressure is not controlled, check her compliance, weight, diet and salt intake. Encourage her to exercise if she is able to do so. She should be gently reminded that she has a 30% risk of a cardiovascular event within 10 years. Combinations of an ACE inhibitor, β-blockers, dihydropyridine calcium-channel blockers, thiazide diuretics and α-blockers are all suitable. It is important to address all cardiovascular risk factors. It is clearly going to be difficult for this patient to achieve her blood pressure targets, and she will need help, encouragement and regular monitoring.

6. Yes, so long as there are no side effects.

FURTHER READING

ALLHAT Officers and Coordinators for the ALLHAT Collaborative Research Group. Major outcomes in high-risk patients randomised to angiotensin-converting-enzyme inhibitor or calcium-channel blocker vs diuretic. The Antihypertensive and Lipid-Lowering Treatment to Prevent Heart Attack Trial (ALLHAT). *JAMA*. 2002; **288:** 2981–97.

August P. Initial treatment of hypertension. *NEJM*. 2003; **348:** 610–17.

Benetos, A, Thomas F, Bean K, *et al.* Prognostic value of systolic and diastolic blood pressure in treated hypertensive men. *Arch Intern Med*. 2002; **162:** 577–81.

Blood Pressure Lowering Treatment Trialists Collaboration. Effects of angiotensin-converting-enzyme inhibitors, calcium antagonists and other blood-pressure-lowering drugs on mortality and major cardiovascular morbidity. *Lancet*. 2000; **356:** 1955–64.

Brown M. Matching the right drug to the right patient in essential hypertension. *Heart*. 2001; **86:** 113–20.

Brown MJ, Palmer CR, Castaigne A, *et al.* Morbidity and mortality in patients randomised to double-blind treatment with once daily calcium channel blockade or diuretic in the International Nifedipine GITS Study: Intervention as a Goal in Hypertension Treatment (INSIGHT). *Lancet*. 2000; **356:** 366–72.

Clement DL, De Buyzere ML, De Bacquer DA, *et al.* Prognostic value of ambulatory blood-pressure recordings in patients with treated hypertension. *NEJM.* 2003; **348:** 2407–15.

Fourth Joint Task Force of the European Society of Cardiology and Other Societies on Cardiovascular Disease Prevention in Clinical Practice (constituted by representatives of nine societies and by invited experts). European guidelines on cardiovascular disease prevention in clinical practice: executive summary. *Eur Heart J.* 2007; **28:** 2375–414.

Franklin SS, Khan SA, Wong ND, *et al.* Is pulse pressure useful in predicting risk for coronary heart disease? The Framingham heart study. *Circulation.* 1999; **100:** 354–60.

Handler C, Coghlan G. *Living with Coronary Disease.* London: Springer; 2007.

Heart Outcomes Prevention Evaluation Study Investigators. Effects of ramipril on cardiovascular and microvascular outcomes in people with diabetes mellitus: results of the HOPE study and MICRO-HOPE substudy. *Lancet.* 2000; **355:** 253–9.

National Collaborating Centre for Chronic Conditions. *Hypertension. Management of hypertension in adults in primary care: partial update.* Update of NICE Clinical Guideline 18 (published in August 2004). London: National Collaborating Centre for Chronic Conditions; 2006.

O'Brien E. Ambulatory blood pressure monitoring in the management of hypertension. *Heart.* 2003; **89:** 571–6.

Pickering T. How common is white coat hypertension? *JAMA.* 1988; **259:** 225–8.

Ramsay LE, Williams B, Johnston GD, *et al.* BHS Guidelines. Guidelines for the management of hypertension: report of the Third Working Party of the British Hypertension Society. *J Hum Hypertens.* 1999; **13:** 569–92.

Van Jaarsveld BC, Krijnen P, Pieterman H, *et al.* The effect of balloon angioplasty on hypertension in atherosclerotic renal-artery stenosis. *NEJM.* 2000; **342:** 1007–14.

Wing LMH, Reid CM, Ryan P, *et al.* A comparison of outcomes with angiotensin-converting-enzyme inhibitors and diuretics for hypertension in the elderly. *NEJM.* 2003; **348:** 583–92.

Lipid disorders and emerging risk factors for cardiovascular disease

FIVE

Clinical cases

1. A 63-year-old man attends your surgery two weeks after leaving hospital following a heart attack. He is slim, a non-smoker and normotensive. In addition to aspirin and atenolol, a statin has been prescribed, and he would like to stop taking it because he has a 'good diet'. What advice do you give him?
2. A 28-year-old woman comes to see you, distressed after the death of her 73-year-old father who died suddenly a few days previously, having had 'high cholesterol'. She wants to know what she should do to avoid the same fate as her father.
3. An 83-year-old hypertensive lady with type 2 diabetes and frequent episodes of angina is brought to your surgery by her daughter who lives with her. What do you do?
4. A 59-year-old man who has been on a statin for six months comes to see you one month after coronary angioplasty complaining of aches in his thighs. What do you do?
5. A 60-year-old retired GP with well-controlled hypertension and diabetes, who is an occasional cigar smoker, asks for advice because his LDL is 4.0, his total cholesterol 5.5 and his triglycerides are 3.2. He was told by one of his ex-patients at the golf club that he should be on a statin and a fibrate. Do you agree?

Management of lipid disorders

A high cholesterol level is the single biggest risk factor for coronary heart disease. The majority of the UK population aged over 50 years has a high cholesterol level. Cholesterol consists mainly of the low-density lipoprotein cholesterol (LDL-C).

Effective lowering of LDL-C and increasing the level of high-density lipoprotein cholesterol (HDL-C), reduces the amount of atheroma in arteries and the risk of both fatal and non-fatal cardiovascular events. The lower the LDL-C level, the greater the effect. These observations have prompted lower targets for cholesterol treatment. For secondary prevention, the Joint British Societies have set targets of <4.0 mmol/l for total cholesterol and <2.0 mmol/l for LDL cholesterol or reducing LDL-C by 30% and cholesterol by 25%, whichever is the lower absolute value.

It is important to have a basic understanding of the physiology of lipids and how treatments are used to lower cholesterol. Managing hyperlipidaemia requires an understanding of:

- lipid physiology
- the patient's absolute coronary risk
- the importance of lipid lowering in primary and secondary prevention
- the patient's lifestyle and other coexisting clinical conditions
- the impact and limitations of lifestyle changes and drugs on lipid levels and other risk factors in long-term risk reduction

❖ lipid-lowering drugs and their adverse effects

❖ practical difficulties of patient adherence to advice and prescribed treatments.

The need for good advice given well

Perhaps most importantly, successful management ultimately depends on how the advice is given and the patient's ability to understand it and make the necessary long-term changes. This highlights the importance of the relationship the patient has with the primary care team and the complex art of giving a patient personal lifestyle advice which is often not requested and occasionally resented.

Treating hyperlipidaemia and hypertension both require similar professional skills and a comprehensive appreciation of cardiovascular risk in different patient groups. Lifestyle changes in these conditions are effective to some degree and should be started before and continuously underpin drug interventions.

Patient variation in compliance with treatment

Patients vary in their willingness to take medication and follow medical advice. Some are very keen to take medication – for example, non-prescribed aspirin to reduce their cardiovascular risk, even though they may be at low risk. Some older patients may consider suggested lifestyle changes or medication as irrelevant or unacceptable. Young patients may take a similar view and feel immune from the distant possibility of a stroke or myocardial infarct. This understandable attitude may also explain the failure of smoking cessation and weight loss programmes in young people. Survivors of infarction and those who have had myocardial revascularisation are usually more compliant, at least initially after the event.

Effective primary and secondary prevention requires the patient to take responsibility for their health but even with enthusiastic education and encouragement, it is unrealistic to expect all patients to maintain compliance in the long term. Reassurance and explanation should be given to patients who are anxious about the safety of long-term medication.

Improving compliance

A large proportion of patients take more than one tablet because they may, in addition to hyperlipidaemia, have hypertension, diabetes and coronary artery disease. Combination tablets and simplified, once-daily doses timed with regular events in patients' daily schedule, improve compliance. Patients, particularly the elderly, may benefit from a visit by a community pharmacist. Family, carers and neighbours often help patients who find it difficult to remember to take their tablets.

It is important to review regularly all the prescribed medication and their doses and ask patients, or those who look after them, whether they take their tablets and if they think they have any resulting side effects. Patients, unless asked, may not wish to upset the doctor by 'confessing' that they do not take their tablets. Patients are more likely to comply with their medication if they understand and agree that they will benefit from it.

What do patients want to know about cholesterol?

They want to know whether they have a high cholesterol level, whether they need to worry about it and why, what food they should avoid, what food or supplements might help, whether they need tablets and, if so, what the side effects might be.

Patients who are slim, exercise frequently and have a low-fat diet may not understand why they have a high cholesterol level. They may know someone who had a heart attack or heart operation who had a 'normal' cholesterol level and may want an explanation as to how this could happen and whether it could happen to them. They may want to know what high- and low-density cholesterol and triglycerides are and what they can do to improve them. What are the 'good' foods to eat and which are the ones they should avoid? Is alcohol good or bad and is red wine really 'good for the heart' and how much should they drink? What foods and drink lower cholesterol? They increasingly ask and expect those who check their blood cholesterol and manage it in primary care to answer these and other questions.

Explaining risk and who needs tablets

Most patients know that a high cholesterol level is bad and may lead to blocked arteries, heart attacks, strokes and furring up in the leg arteries. The higher the cholesterol level, the greater the risk of cardiac events. Conversely, the lower the cholesterol level, the lower the likelihood of these problems. Those tested and shown to have a 'normal' cholesterol level will be pleased and relieved to learn that they have 'passed' the test and so can carry on with their usual lifestyle. Those with hyperlipidaemia may be at low risk from cardiovascular events and may not need medication. In contrast, patients with a 'normal' cholesterol level may be at high absolute cardiovascular risk. This may be confusing and patients will need a clear explanation about this and why the cholesterol level is not the sole determinant for medical treatment.

What are lipoproteins?

Lipoproteins are large molecules that transport cholesterol and triglycerides in the blood. They have a lipid core consisting of triglycerides and cholesterol esters, which is surrounded by phospholipids and apolipoproteins. They are classified according to their density and there are five components:

* chylomicrons are the largest and contain the highest concentration of lipid
* very-low-density lipoproteins (VLDL) made in the liver
* intermediate-density lipoproteins (IDL)
* low-density lipoproteins (LDL) made in the plasma
* high-density lipoproteins (HDL), which are the smallest and contain the least amount of lipids.

About 70% of the plasma total cholesterol is carried in the LDL fraction and 25% in the HDL fraction.

LDL moves cholesterol into the tissues and arteries. Atherogenesis is produced mainly by LDL-C. HDL removes excess cholesterol from cells in the tissues. HDL-C is protective against atherosclerosis.

Cholesterol metabolism and homeostasis

There are two main sources of cholesterol – dietary and that produced by the liver. Most people in developed countries consume 0.3 g of cholesterol per day, and synthesize 1.0 g per day. Cholesterol has to be transported through the blood to the liver for processing, degradation and secretion into bile.

Cholesterol homeostasis is controlled in the liver by a feedback loop controlled by LDL receptors which are increased (up-regulated) and decreased (down-regulated) depending on the amount of cholesterol in the liver cells.

Excess absorbed cholesterol reaching the liver is repackaged and secreted back into the blood as very-low-density lipoproteins (VLDL) and LDL.

Individuals react differently to dietary fat. In two-thirds of normal individuals, the cholesterol level increases very little or not at all despite a cholesterol-rich diet. The blood-cholesterol level in the remainder increases due to cholesterol absorption.

Dietary cholesterol mixes in the bowel lumen with about 900 mg of biliary cholesterol manufactured and secreted by the liver. This is then digested to form free cholesterol, fatty acids and mono- and diglycerides which, through the detergent effects of bile acids, become part of micelles that are transported to absorption sites in the gut lumen. Fifty per cent of this free cholesterol in the gut lumen is absorbed and so a lot of the biliary cholesterol is recycled back to the liver.

All the triglyceride content is absorbed through the gut wall. Only 50% of the cholesterol is absorbed; the remainder is excreted. Cholesterol esters are reconstructed to cholesterol in the gut luminal cells through the action of the enzyme acyl coenzyme A cholesterol acyltransferase (ACAT) and incorporated with triglyceride with 1% protein to become chylomicrons. Chylomicrons are formed after a fatty meal and then transported to the thoracic duct and to the bloodstream via the left subclavian vein. As they pass through the circulation, triglyceride 'fuel' is deposited in striated and cardiac muscle and adipose tissue. The cholesterol ester-containing remnant is highly atherogenic and under normal circumstances is rapidly assimilated by the liver.

Transport of lipids is mainly by the VLDL lipoprotein constructed and secreted by the liver. Lipoprotein lipase extracts the triglyceride leaving behind the atherogenic LDL. The LDL is extracted from the plasma by LDL receptors on the liver cells. Cholesterol is synthesised by the liver and is influenced by LDL receptors in the liver through a negative feedback loop. When intracellular cholesterol levels fall, the LDL receptors are activated and cholesterol is drawn into the liver cells from the circulation for the production of more VLDL and bile acids. Conversely, the higher the cholesterol level in the liver, the lower the production of LDL receptors.

Therefore, cholesterol homeostasis depends upon absorption of cholesterol from the gut through the intestinal mucosal cells and on hepatocyte cells, which control the rate of cholesterol extraction from the plasma into the liver.

New cholesterol drugs have been produced to reduce dietary and biliary cholesterol absorption across the intestinal wall without affecting the absorption of triglycerides and fat-soluble vitamins. An example of this type of drug is ezetimibe.

Cholesterol and atheroma plaque formation

Cholesterol is an essential component of cell membranes, steroid-based hormones (for example, sex hormones), and bile acids produced by the liver. It is the main constituent of atheroma which is deposited inside arterial walls and forms plaques.

Atheroma starts with inflammation and damage to the endothelial surface of the intima of arteries. White cells – monocytes – take up oxidised LDL-C to become macrophage-derived foam cells to form 'fatty streaks' which can be seen by the naked eye lining the artery. There is also proliferation of vascular smooth muscle cells and fibrous tissue. Accumulation of LDL-C and inflammatory cells form the core of an atheromatous plaque. Plaques containing a lot of lipid and which have only a thin fibrous cap are more likely to crack or rupture ('vulnerable plaques') causing heart attacks and strokes. Plaques with less lipid in their core and which have a thick fibrous plaque, are less likely to rupture and are called 'stable plaques'. Therefore, acute coronary syndromes and myocardial infarction occur where the plaque is soft and inflamed and not necessarily at the site of a major stenosis where the plaque might be stable. This pathological observation underlines the low predictive accuracy of calcium scoring imaging methods (electron beam computed tomography) for prognosis.

Plaque rupture

Under certain circumstances, the cap or top covering of these plaques may rupture, exposing the arterial wall. This leads to platelet aggregation and thrombus formation as part of the healing mechanism. In a heart artery, this may result (unless the clot is broken down or dissolved by the body's own thrombolytic processes) in a heart attack. The deposition of cholesterol in arterial walls results in similar problems in the cerebral arteries and leads to impaired blood and oxygen supply to the legs (claudication).

Risks of hypercholesterolaemia

There is a strong graded relationship between a total cholesterol level greater than 4.6 mmol/l and coronary heart disease.

The protective effect of high-density lipoprotein cholesterol is probably as potent as the atherogenic effect of low-density lipoprotein cholesterol, particularly in women.

Benefits of cholesterol reduction

Several trials have shown that reducing cholesterol levels reduce fatal and non-fatal myocardial infarction without increasing death from other causes. An 11% reduction in total cholesterol is associated with a 23% decrease in cardiovascular events. However, even a strict low-fat diet may result in only a 5% reduction in total cholesterol.

Lowering cholesterol slows the natural progression of coronary artery disease and may also 'clear' affected heart arteries – resulting in regression of atheroma. Cardiac event rates have also been reduced out of proportion to the usually small improvements in the angiographic appearances. The benefits of statins result from effects in addition to reducing the bulk of atheroma in arteries.

LDL cholesterol (LDL-C)

The LDL-C level accounts almost entirely for the positive correlation between cholesterol and coronary heart disease. It is atherogenic. Reductions in LDL-C reduce the risk of coronary heart disease. The lower the LDL-C, the lower the risk of cardiovascular events.

> Every 1.0 mmol/l reduction in LDL-C is associated with a 12% decrease in all cause mortality, a 19% decrease in coronary mortality and a 19% decrease in stroke, independent of the starting level of LDL-C.
> The lower the LDL, the better.

A target level of <1.8 mmol/l is recommended by many cardiologists for secondary prevention. However, even at this low level in patients treated with statins, there remains a 20% five-year risk of a major cardiovascular event (compared with a 25% risk in the untreated patients) in patients with vascular disease.

The minimum concentration of LDL-C required for atherogenesis in man appears to be 2 mmol/l. The relative risk of coronary heart disease is <2, with an LDL-C level of <4 mmol/l, and 35 in patients with familial hypercholesterolaemia and an LDL-C level of >6 mmol/l. Therefore, a slight increase in LDL-C increases risk disproportionately and substantially.

HDL cholesterol (HDL-C)

A high HDL level is protective, probably by reversing cholesterol transport away from the vessel wall and transporting it to the liver. It may also reduce inflammation and act as an antioxidant reducing LDL-C deposition in the artery. This might produce regression of atheroma.

From epidemiological observations, HDL-C is a stronger predictor of risk than LDL-C. Each 1% *increase* in LDL-C increases risk by 1%, whereas each 1% *decrease* in HDL-C increases risk by 3%.

A level of <1 mmol/l is considered 'low' and a level above 1.5 is 'high'. There is currently no evidence from trials that increasing HDL levels decreases cardiovascular risk.

Low HDL levels are associated with obesity, physical inactivity, severe renal failure, type 2 diabetes and cigarette smoking. Thiazides and β-blockers reduce HDL levels. There are no guidelines for managing patients with a low HDL level which is an independent risk factor for coronary heart disease.

Vigorous sustained exercise (for example, long-distance running), and moderate alcohol consumption are associated with high HDL levels. Nicotinic acid is the most effective drug in increasing HDL-C.

Recently, toracetrapib, a cholesterol ester transfer protein inhibitor, which increases HDL-C by 60%, was withdrawn from use after a trial comparing it with atorvastatin showed an increased mortality associated with toracetrapib.

A low HDL-C level appears to be more important as an adverse risk factor than a high HDL-C level being protective. An effective approach would be to increase HDL-C and lower LDL-C. However, there is insufficient evidence to recommend drugs to increase HDL levels.

Triglycerides

Triglycerides are made in the liver and transported with cholesterol as VLDL. Together with cholesterol as part of absorbed dietary fat, they constitute chylomicrons.

The most important clinical consequences of a high triglyceride level are coronary artery disease, cerebrovascular disease and peripheral vascular disease. Acute pancreatitis is a rare consequence of extremely high levels. No trials have been performed to determine whether decreasing triglycerides in isolation from other lipids reduces cardiovascular risk. Measuring triglycerides alone for estimation of cardiovascular risk has no advantage over measuring total cholesterol. Most laboratories include triglyceride levels in the lipid profile.

Aggressive lipid lowering with statins may have effects other than cholesterol lowering. These include:

- stabilising atheromatous plaques by depleting them of the soft 'explosive' lipid core, thus making them less liable to rupture
- stabilising the endothelium
- inhibiting platelet aggregation
- modifying the behaviour of vascular smooth muscle cells.

These effects support the increasing use of statins in patients with vascular disease in any arterial territory and those with high LDL levels with or without a high total cholesterol level.

Similar beneficial effects have also been found with statin treatment in patients with carotid artery disease. Carotid artery intimal thickening (an early stage of atheroma) and cerebrovascular events are reduced.

Risk factors for vascular disease

At least 80% of major coronary heart disease events in middle-aged men can be attributed to the three strongest risk factors – smoking, hypertension and serum total cholesterol.

Cardiovascular risk factors may be classified as:
✧ major independent risk factors
✧ life habit risk factors
✧ emerging risk factors.

Major risk factors
✧ Age.
✧ Cigarette smoking.
✧ Hypertension (BP>140/90 mmHg).
✧ HDL <1 mmol/l.
✧ Raised LDL >3.0 mmol/l.
✧ Family history of premature coronary artery disease (first-degree male relative <55 years or female relative <65 years).
✧ Renal impairment.

These established major risk factors account for, individually or in combination, most cardiovascular disease.

Life-habit risk factors
✧ Obesity.
✧ Physical inactivity.
✧ Atherogenic diet.

Emerging risk factors
✧ Homocysteine.
✧ Lipoprotein (a).
✧ Prothrombotic factors and fibrinogen.
✧ Proinflammatory factors (C reactive protein – CRP).
✧ Impaired fasting glucose.
✧ Subclinical atherosclerosis.
✧ Stress.
✧ Social class.

None of the emerging risk factors add substantially to risk assessment or predicting cardiovascular events.

Measuring lipid levels – random or fasting?

Although total and HDL cholesterol levels are not significantly influenced by a fatty meal, it is sensible to advise patients to have a fasting blood sample. The laboratory may not measure the HDL directly but estimate it from the LDL level which is affected by a recent meal containing fat.

Risk assessment

Count the major risk factors. If there are two or more, perform a 10-year absolute coronary risk assessment. Patients with no more than one risk factor are at low risk and would probably have a 10-year coronary risk of <10% and would not benefit significantly from drug interventions.

Principles of interventions in primary and secondary prevention

Patients with known vascular disease (previous infarct, revascularisation and peripheral vascular disease, cerebrovascular disease) are at high risk (10-year risk of a cardiovascular event is >20%) and so the threshold for initiating lifestyle and drug treatment is lower. LDL goal levels should be lower (<2.5 mmol/l) and these patients should be treated with a statin. Fibrates and nicotinic acid are used in addition for patients with raised triglycerides.

In contrast, *patients at low risk (10-year risk <10%) should be encouraged to take primary preventative measures and would not usually need drug intervention unless their LDL >4.8 mmol/l.*

Should we lower cholesterol as much as possible?

There is considerable debate about this. The American National Education Program recommends lowering LDL cholesterol to less than 1.8 mmol/l, which is difficult to achieve even with very big doses of statin. This would put most of the western world's adult population on a big dose of a statin with the associated increased risk of adverse effects. Although a high dose of atorvastatin (80 mg) reduced cardiovascular events by 22% compared with conventional doses, mortality was not reduced. Side effects are more likely with very high doses of statins.

At present it appears reasonable to continue to lower lipid levels aggressively in those most at risk who have cardiovascular disease and a high risk of further cardiovascular complications.

Health economics: influence of resources on guidelines

If statins cost the same as aspirin, a primary prevention case could be made for treating even 'low'-risk individuals (10-year risk <10%), although there may be a risk of side effects. Patients with a 10-year risk as low as 6% would derive prognostic benefit from statins, with a reduction in coronary events and deaths from all causes. It has been estimated that this would entail treating nearly 60% of the UK population. Lowering the threshold for using statins has enormous cost implications in the UK because of the way most drugs are licensed and dispensed. Generic statins are available 'over the counter' in the UK and in other countries, so that patients can make their own decision about whether they want to take them.

Variations in guideline recommendations

National guidelines formulated by the Joint British Societies make useful evidence-based recommendations for starting treatment for primary and secondary cardiovascular prevention.

Financial considerations influence treatment thresholds, which vary considerably between different countries and depend largely on medication and implementation costs. The scientific evidence shows statins improve prognosis in people with a 10-year cardiovascular risk of 10%. The Joint British Societies recommend statins only when the risk exceeds 15%; the Joint European Task Force on Coronary Heart Disease at 20%, and the NHS framework on cardiovascular disease prevention at a risk of 30%. The US National Cholesterol Education Program (NCEP) recommendations use lower thresholds.

Most GPs use the Joint British Societies' Recommendations, which will be updated. The thresholds for using statins are partially set by NHS financial restraints. The current thresholds for initiating statins may well be lowered in future and this may bring them in line with the USA guidelines published by the National Heart Lung and Blood Institute (NHLBI).

Summary of Joint British Societies' Recommendations

The aim of cardiovascular prevention is to reduce the risk of non-fatal or fatal atherosclerotic cardiac events and to improve both quality and length of life. This should be done through lifestyle and risk-factor interventions and where necessary, drugs to reduce blood pressure, lipids, and normalise the blood sugar.

The current guidelines recommend treating all people who are at high risk equally:
1. people with atherosclerotic cardiovascular disease in any territory
2. diabetics
3. apparently healthy individuals at high risk (>20% over 10 years).

❖ Total cholesterol level of <5 mmol/l and LDL <3.0 mmol/l for primary prevention; a total cholesterol level of <4 mmol/l and LDL level of <2.5 mmol/l for secondary prevention. Sixty per cent of the population have a level greater than this. If, despite lifestyle and dietary changes, the absolute coronary risk remains above 15% and the total cholesterol is greater than 5.0 mmol/l, start a statin or, if the triglycerides are raised in addition, a fibrate.

✧ Calculate 10-year coronary heart disease risk using Joint British Societies' assessment chart prior to lifestyle changes or treatment. All cardiovascular risk factors should be addressed.

✧ Secondary causes of hyperlipidaemia should be corrected.

✧ Diabetics should be given a statin if their 10-year coronary heart disease risk exceeds 15%.

✧ Fibrates should be used if triglyceride levels >2.3 mmol/l despite lipid-lowering diet.

✧ Lipoprotein analysis should include fasting total cholesterol, total triglycerides and HDL levels. The LDL can be calculated thus:

$$LDL = TC - (TG/2.19 + HDL)$$

Note: The terms 'high' and 'low' cardiovascular risk are artificial and arbitrary. They have different meanings for the patient, the doctor and a statistician. A middle-aged patient told that he had a 9% risk of dying from a heart attack within 10 years may feel that this is not 'low' risk. An octogenarian, on the other hand, given the same prognosis, may feel quite reassured. Guidelines for cardiovascular risk reduction should be interpreted and applied with an understanding of the patient's clinical condition, their overall risk profile and an appreciation of their wishes.

The following four points are not detailed in the Joint British Societies' Recommendations.

✧ All patients (both primary and secondary prevention) should have 'lifestyle advice'.

✧ Diabetics are at high risk and the target blood pressure is lower.

✧ Patients with cardiovascular risk equivalents are not specified in the current Joint British Societies' Recommendations.

✧ 'Targeting progressively more patients' underlines the uncertainty of treating patients at intermediate risk.

Priorities for cardiovascular risk management

First priority: patients with established coronary artery disease or other atherosclerotic disease (secondary prevention)

✧ Relevant lifestyle changes: stopping smoking, increasing exercise, eating healthier food.

✧ Blood pressure controlled to below 140/85 mmHg.

✧ Diabetes: optimal control of blood glucose; target BP <130/80 mmHg (although this is often not possible); reduce total cholesterol to <5.0 mmol/l and LDL cholesterol to <3.0 mmol/l.

✧ Cardioprotective drugs for 'selected' patients: aspirin, ACE inhibitors, β-blockers, statins.

Second priority: patients without known coronary heart disease or other atherosclerotic disease (primary prevention)

There are three groups to be identified and managed in a staged approach – the group with the highest risk first. All patients should be given relevant lifestyle advice.

1. Absolute 10-year CHD risk of >30%.
⋄ Blood pressure controlled to <140/85 mmHg.
⋄ Reduce total cholesterol to <5.0 mmol/l and LDL<3.0 mmol/l.
⋄ Diabetes: optimal control of blood glucose, blood pressure to 140/80 mmHg.
⋄ Aspirin for patients >50 years if male and/or hypertensive.

2. Absolute 10-year CHD risk of >15%
⋄ 'Target progressively more patients' and intervene as described above.

3. Absolute 10-year CHD risk of <15%
⋄ Drug treatment is not required unless there is hypertension >160/100 mmHg with associated target organ damage or familial hyperlipidaemia.

Cardiovascular risk equivalents

Patients with the following conditions are at equivalent cardiovascular risk to those who have coronary artery disease and should be screened. They should be considered for statins irrespective of their lipid levels.
⋄ Known vascular disease (coronary, cerebrovascular, peripheral).
⋄ Hypertension.
⋄ Abdominal aortic aneurysm.
⋄ Diabetes.
⋄ Transient ischaemic attacks.
⋄ Previous stroke.

Hypertensive patients, particularly men over 60 years of age, should be examined for an abdominal aortic aneurysm and have an ultrasound if necessary. Feel the foot pulses in all patients with claudication, hypertension and diabetes. Duplex ultrasound should be performed if patients have symptoms.

Causes of secondary hyperlipidaemia

Most patients with hyperlipidaemia have a 'primary' or genetic cause. The 'secondary' causes below should be considered and, where necessary, treated. This may result in a substantial improvement in the lipid profile and make drug treatment for the hyperlipidaemia unnecessary. Tight control of diabetes and correction of hypothyroidism improve the lipid profile. Both β-blockers and thiazides have an unfavourable effect on lipids and this should be considered in patients with hypertension and hyperlipidaemia.

TABLE 5.1 Causes of secondary hyperlipidaemia and their effect on lipids

DISORDER	CHOLESTEROL	TRIGLYCERIDES	HDL
Hypothyroidism	++	–	–
Type 2 diabetes	+	++	–
Renal disease	++	++	–
Obstructive liver disease	++	–	–
Alcohol	++	++	+
Thiazide	+	+	–
β-blockers	+	+	–
Anorexia nervosa	+++	–	–

Key: – no effect, + mild increase, ++ moderate increase, +++ major increase

Family history

A family history of death from coronary heart disease in either parent before the age of 55 doubles an individual's risk of fatal and non-fatal myocardial infarction. The effect of family history as a risk factor is largely independent of other risk factors implying a separate mechanism.

Hypertension

There is a strong and graded relation between blood pressure and cardiovascular disease, but no clear threshold value which separates hypertensive patients who will experience future cardiovascular events from those who will not.

Diabetes

This is an important, common and modifiable cardiovascular risk factor. Diabetics should have comprehensive risk-factor assessment. The treatment goal is for normal blood sugar levels and correction of other modifiable risk factors. Diabetics have a high mortality both during and after acute myocardial infarction. The short- and long-term results of myocardial revascularisation with both angioplasty and coronary artery bypass are worse for diabetic patients than for non-diabetic patients.

Statins should be prescribed in diabetic patients with a coronary heart disease risk of >15%.

Smoking

The risk of cardiovascular disease is proportional to the number of cigarettes smoked and how deeply the smoker inhales. The risks of pipe and cigar smokers are intermediate compared with the risks of non-smokers and cigarette smokers.

Renal impairment

Minor renal impairment is as powerful a cardiovascular risk factor as diabetes. Patients with cardiovascular disease and impaired renal function are a high-risk subgroup.

Chronic kidney disease with a minor elevation in serum creatinine is associated with an increased cardiovascular risk including cardiovascular death, myocardial infarction and stroke. Impaired renal function independently increases the risk of death in hypertensive patients. Even minor renal impairment adversely affects the outcome of patients with acute coronary syndromes, myocardial infarction and the results of angioplasty and coronary artery surgery.

Microalbuminuria

The levels of albumin in normal people and in disease states, and the albumin : creatinine ratios for men and woman are shown in Table 5.2.

TABLE 5.2 Subdivisions of protein detected in the urine

URINE EXAMINATION	24-HOUR URINARY ALBUMIN EXCRETION (MG)	ALBUMIN : CREATININE RATIO
Normal	<30	<2.5 men; <3.5 women
Microalbuminuria	30–300	2.5–25 men; 3.5–25 women
Macroalbuminuria	>300	>25 men; >25 women

Microalbuminuria is therefore not a disease but describes, like other risk variables, a continuum, like hypertension. Microalbuminuria is three times more common in diabetics, hypertensives and those with enlarged hearts compared with those without any of these conditions. Its presence predicts the development of proteinuria and end-stage renal disease, as well as cardiovascular disease. The proposed atherogenic mechanisms include chronic vascular inflammation, a prothrombotic state and endothelial damage. There is no evidence, however, that reducing proteinuria reduces cardiovascular risk.

Albuminuria is as important a risk factor as smoking, or an increase in total cholesterol of 2 mmol/l, tripling the risk of cardiovascular death, and increasing all-risk mortality by 48%. These effects are independent of renal function, hypertension or diabetes.

Microalbuminuria is a marker of generalised vascular dysfunction, and an important independent risk factor for acute cardiac events and death.

Microalbuminuria and diabetes

Microalbuminuria predicts the development of type 2 diabetes mellitus in 25% of patients. Diabetics with microalbuminuria may progress to macroalbuminuria and end-stage renal disease.

Controlling diabetes reduces microalbuminuria and macro- and microvascular diabetic complications.

> In diabetics, hypertensives, the obese, and those with the metabolic syndrome, microalbuminuria is a marker of poor prognosis due to cardiovascular and renal complications.

ECG abnormalities

Major ECG changes

Q-waves, ST-segment depression and deep ischaemic T-wave inversion suggest important coronary artery disease and are markers as powerful as high cholesterol level, diabetes or hypertension in predicting subsequent cardiac events. Q-waves are the most reliable sign of previous myocardial infarction and coronary artery disease.

Minor ECG changes

These include non-specific ST-segment and minor T-wave flattening or mild inversion. These, too, are associated with a poor prognosis and a higher risk of cardiovascular events compared to patients with a normal ECG.

> Recording an ECG as part of cardiovascular risk assessment is valuable. ECG abnormalities are a risk factor for cardiovascular events and ECG abnormalities may occur silently.

Angiotensin-converting enzyme (ACE) inhibitors and angiotensin II receptor blockers

Angiotensin II damages the kidneys by altering intrarenal haemodynamics, and damages the glomeruli, partly by increasing glomerular capillary permeability. Pharmacological blockade of the renin–angiotensin system reduces cardiovascular risk in patients with renal impairment, and prevents progressive renal disease in diabetics.

ACE inhibitors reduce cardiovascular death, myocardial infarction, and stroke in patients with vascular disease but without heart failure (relative risk reduction of 18%).

Part of the reason that ACE inhibitors and angiotensin II receptor blockers may have superior cardiovascular effects (stroke reduction) in hypertensives compared to β-blockers, is because of their actions on reducing angiotensin II levels and reducing microalbuminuria, through their actions on vascular endothelium.

In type 2 diabetes, ACE inhibitors and angiotensin II receptor antagonists are superior to calcium antagonists and β-blockers in reducing proteinuria and progression of renal disease. Both drugs can be used together synergistically. There is no corresponding reduction in mortality.

Angiotensin-converting enzyme inhibitors should not be withheld from patients with cardiovascular disease because of mild renal impairment. Angiotensin-converting enzyme inhibitors may increase the serum creatinine but should be continued with monitoring of renal function and the dose reduced only if there are major increases in serum creatinine. Their beneficial effects against heart failure in patients with acute myocardial infarction are greater in patients with more severe renal impairment and their efficacy is enhanced with β-blockers.

Exercise

Lifestyle interventions are important and effective components in primary and secondary prevention of coronary artery disease and atheromatous vascular disease in general. Regular aerobic (cardiovascular) exercise has an important and graded effect in reducing cardiovascular mortality. Sedentary individuals have a 1.6 greater relative risk compared with highly active individuals. Exercise has a beneficial effect on blood pressure and serum lipids by reducing triglycerides and has a modest effect in reducing LDL and in increasing HDL levels. Conversely, lack of exercise increases the risk of coronary heart disease and cardiovascular mortality.

Maintenance of a low-fat, low-calorie diet and regular exercise programme is very difficult but important and helpful, particularly in secondary prevention. Primary and secondary prevention clinics should be offered to patients (particularly high-risk patients) and are likely to be successful if run by enthusiastic, well-informed staff.

Obesity

Obesity is an independent risk factor for cardiovascular disease and may have more prognostic importance in women than in men, and in young rather than in old people. Central obesity is measured using the waist : hip ratio and this is a better predictor than overall adiposity such as body mass index.

Obesity is positively correlated with fasting triglyceride and cholesterol levels.

Alcohol

Mild to moderate alcohol consumption reduces the risk of cardiovascular disease and there is an inverse relationship between alcohol and death from coronary heart disease. Moderate alcohol consumption may potentiate the protective cardiovascular benefits of daily exercise.

Taking more than two units of alcohol per day may increase the risk of death from cancer and cirrhosis. Alcohol is fattening. There is no convincing evidence that red wine is superior to other types of alcohol. There is no evidence from controlled trials showing that alcohol reduces total mortality. There is insufficient evidence to encourage patients who do not drink alcohol to start.

Left ventricular hypertrophy

This is a common result of hypertension and a strong predictor of cardiovascular events particularly when associated with a repolarisation change on the electrocardiogram.

Vascular inflammation

Inflammation is believed to be an important step in atherosclerosis and plaque rupture leading to acute coronary syndromes. There is debate about whether C-reactive protein (CRP) is a bystander or a contributor to atherosclerosis.

Homocysteine

In 1959 it was recognised that patients with homocysteinuria developed vascular abnormalities. High levels of homocysteine are a weak but independent risk factor for the development of vascular atherosclerotic disorders and thromboembolic disease. The concentration of homocysteine is inversely related to that of folate and vitamins B_{12} and B_6. High levels may also increase platelet aggregation and damage vascular endothelium. Increases of 5 μmol/L have been associated with significant increases in coronary heart disease but after adjusting for confounding variables, the association is not convincing.

The normal range of homocysteine in the blood is unclear. Levels are higher in males and patients with renal impairment and rise with age and deficiencies of folate and vitamin B_{12}. Homocysteine may be spuriously raised if blood is stored at room temperature. Measuring it is time consuming and expensive and currently not widely available or requested.

Folate is present in green leafy vegetables. Folate treatment in a dose of 0.8 mg per day can reduce the homocysteine level by 25%.

Although there is some laboratory and clinical evidence for considering homocysteine as a potential risk factor for coronary artery disease, there is as yet no evidence that reducing homocysteine with folate reduces vascular morbidity or mortality.

> Screening for homocysteinuria for either primary or secondary prevention with a view to treatment with folic acid is not recommended.

Lipoprotein (a)

Discovered in 1963 and synthesised in the liver, lipoprotein (a) consists of an LDL particle linked to a molecule of apo (a) protein, which is a large protein similar to plasminogen.

Concentrations increase with LDL cholesterol levels, are higher in Afro-Caribbeans than in Caucasians and in all patients with renal disease, diabetics and after myocardial infarction. High levels of lipoprotein (a) combined with high LDL levels have been associated with a high risk of coronary artery disease but this is not consistent and the mechanism is unknown. It is not clear whether it is an independent risk factor or whether reducing levels of lipo (a) reduce cardiovascular events. Therefore, lipoprotein (a) is not routinely measured.

Fibrinogen and other haemostatic markers

Fibrinogen is a key component of a fibrin clot, platelet aggregation and blood viscosity. Fibrinogen levels are raised in patients after myocardial infarction. Fibrinogen is synthesised in the liver. Levels are higher in women than in men; higher in smokers; increase with age, alcohol consumption, renal impairment, glucose intolerance; increase after the menopause and with obesity.

Stress at work has been shown to be associated with raised levels of fibrinogen. Levels are reduced with weight loss, reduced alcohol consumption, exercise, and bezafibrate and platelet inhibitors. A fibrinogen concentration of >3.1 g/l is associated with relative risks of coronary heart disease of 1.6 in men and 2.9 in women.

It is not routinely measured and at present there are no specific fibrinogen-lowering drugs.

Other prothrombotic factors have been investigated but their prognostic importance is unclear. Tissue plasminogen activator inhibitor-1 and D-dimer may be associated with increased cardiovascular events. Factor VIIc has an inverse association. Fibrinogen and factor VII are strongly correlated with triglycerides and hypercoagulability. These markers are not routinely measured in clinical practice.

Brain natriuretic peptide (BNP)

BNP has been shown to predict cardiovascular events in patients with angina.

Role or biomarkers in predicting cardiovascular events

Although novel markers of thrombogenicity and inflammation, chronic infection and oxidative stress may be associated with atherosclerosis, they do not appear to provide significantly more prognostic information in identifying patients at risk of cardiovascular events. Therefore, most information is derived from conventional risk factors.

Chlamydia pneumoniae

Although it was proposed that previous infection with *Chlamydia pneumoniae* increased the risk of coronary artery disease, subsequent studies have shown that there is no convincing association.

Dietary recommendations for patients with hyperlipidaemia

The general principle is to eat as little fat as possible – preferably none at all. Some patients may appreciate referral to a dietician and this should be discussed with the patient. Patients, not surprisingly, get very confused after being given complicated advice including the percentages of saturated fat (<7%), polyunsaturated fat (<10%), mono-unsaturated fat (<20%) and total fat (30%) of their total calorie intake together with less than 200 g of cholesterol per day.

How one measures these amounts is difficult for medical staff to understand and explain! The simpler the advice, the more likely the patient is to follow it. You may wish to give patients a list of fatty foods which they should avoid completely.

Oat bran 50–100 g per day and soya protein 25 g per day each reduce total cholesterol by 2–3%.

One portion of oily fish per week is recommended because it contains omega-3 fatty acids, which are protective against coronary heart disease, reduce susceptibility to cardiac arrhythmia, blood clotting and plasma triglycerides. Omega-3 fatty acids are thought to protect against fatal myocardial infarction and sudden death. This is supported by the low risk of coronary heart disease-related death in Japan where the national diet includes a lot of raw oily fish.

In a large cohort of post-menopausal women, a low-fat diet had only modest effects on cardiovascular risk factors and did not result in decreased cardiac events over a period of eight years. However, a Mediterranean diet in high-risk patients lowered risk factors more effectively than a conventional low-fat diet.

Hormone replacement treatment (HRT) in women – effect on lipids

Observational studies showed that HRT might protect women against coronary heart disease but randomised clinical trials have not confirmed this.

Hormone replacement therapy does not protect women against death, coronary heart disease or myocardial infarction. In diabetic women, HRT significantly increases the risk of death from all causes and coronary heart disease. The reasons are unclear.

Oestrogens increase triglycerides, particularly when given orally, and may occasionally precipitate acute pancreatitis and so should be avoided in women with very high triglycerides levels. These should be checked before starting treatment. Patch oestrogen may need to be given because this has little effect on triglycerides levels. Oestrogen reduces LDL cholesterol and increases HDL cholesterol.

Stress

Job strain and effort-reward imbalance increase cardiovascular mortality. One possible mechanism is that high stress levels (low salary, low job control, lack of social approval and few career opportunities) are associated with hypertension, raised LDL cholesterol levels and raised fibrinogen levels and reduced fibrinolytic activity. High work stress levels resulting from 'organisational injustice' are associated with low heart rate variability and increased catecholamine levels. Although stress at work may double the risk of cardiovascular death among employees, there is, as yet, no evidence that stress reduction decreases this risk.

Other psychological characteristics – depression, anxiety, anger, type-A personality and hostility – have also been suggested as cardiovascular risk factors. There is increasing evidence that severe anxiety is a robust and independent risk factor for myocardial infarction among older men. Depression is recognised as a risk factor for cardiovascular disease. Severe anxiety may trigger myocardial infarction and is well recognised as a precipitating factor for angina, presumably due to increased heart rate and blood pressure.

Social class

The mortality from coronary heart disease is lower and decreasing more quickly in social class I compared with that in social class V. The reasons for this are unclear, but are probably multifactorial – including diet, exercise, smoking and obesity.

Treating the elderly

Coronary heart disease is the leading cause of death in elderly patients with more than 80% of coronary deaths occurring in patients over the age of 65 (although this would not now be considered elderly). Statins are used in around 40–60% of patients after myocardial infarction and this is generally believed to be suboptimal.

In elderly patients with coronary heart disease, statins reduce all cause mortality by 22%, coronary disease mortality by 30%, non-fatal myocardial infarction by 26%, the need for revascularisation by 30%, and stroke by 30%. The number needed to treat and the absolute risk reduction in the elderly is, compared with younger patients, relatively small at 60.

> Reducing non-fatal major adverse cardiac events and stroke is important in the elderly because this reduces functional decline and permanent disability.

Although lipid trials have excluded patients aged over 75 years, it is accepted that patients older than this with established coronary artery disease should be managed in the same way as younger patients. Statins should be used where appropriate in full consultation with the patient. An ageist approach is likely to be resented by fit octogenarians with symptomatic vascular disease. The decision to start a statin in a symptom-free pensioner with an isolated raised LDL level is more difficult and their views about wanting to avoid their first and possibly final heart attack should be respected.

Ethnic risks

South Asians have a 50% greater risk of developing coronary heart disease compared with Caucasian people living in the UK, while Afro-Caribbeans have a lower risk. South Asians are at greater risk from cardiovascular disease and have a tendency to have a low HDL, high triglycerides, diabetes, obesity and hypertension (metabolic syndrome). Coronary artery disease tends to more diffuse and the arteries appear to be smaller possibly because there is widespread vascular disease.

> It has been estimated that >60% of primary coronary events could be prevented by adoption of a healthy lifestyle (defined as regular exercise, no smoking, attainment of ideal weight, moderate alcohol consumption, and a healthy diet).

Drug therapy for lipid disorders

Lipid treatment is usually for life. Warn the patient about potential side effects of all drugs before prescribing. Not all symptoms are side effects.

Statins

Statins specifically inhibit hydroxymethyl-glutaryl coenzyme A reductase (HMG CoA reductase) – the rate-limiting step in cholesterol synthesis. They have made a major impact in treating patients with, and those at risk of, vascular disease. They reduce VLDL and LDL concentrations and induction of the LDL receptors. The major effect of statins is reducing LDL cholesterol although atorvastatin reduces triglycerides as well. Statins are more effective than other drugs in reducing LDL-cholesterol but less effective than fibrates in reducing triglycerides.

Statins have several possible modes of action apart from reducing LDL levels. These include a direct effect on endothelial function, reducing the inflammatory reactions (CRP levels fall) and changes in arteries, plaque stabilisation, and reducing thrombus formation.

Adverse effects of statins

They are generally well tolerated and are the most effective lipid-lowering drugs. The most common side effects are headache, gastrointestinal side effects, abdominal pain and bloating, flatulence and nausea. Rash and hypersensitivity are very unusual. They do not increase morbidity or mortality, nor do they increase the risk of cancer.

Statins should be used with caution in patients with a history of liver disease or a high alcohol intake. Liver function tests should be carried out before and within three months after starting treatment and then 6–12 months after. Statins occasionally cause disturbed liver function tests and should be stopped if the serum transaminase level rises persistently to three times the upper limit of normal. Patients should be advised to report unexplained muscle pains.

Only very rarely (four cases in 100 000 patient years after atorvastatin) do statins cause myopathy sufficient to cause rhabdomyolysis and myoglobinuria and death from renal failure. Myalgia, myositis and myopathy have been reported. If myopathy is suspected, check the creatine kinase level. If this is raised to five times the normal level, stop the statin. The risk of myopathy is increased if the patient is also taking a fibrate or cyclosporine.

Results of statins

A response is seen within four weeks. If patients cannot tolerate them, try a different statin or one of the other group of drugs discussed below, which may be used together with a statin, in patients with persistently high lipid levels or in patients with a high-risk profile. Doubling the dose of statin to the recommended maximum achieves a modest lowering of the LDL and total cholesterol. Although some physicians prescribe statins to be taken at night to slow down the endogenous cholesterol pathway, which may be more active at night (it may be suppressed during the day by fatty meals), the timing of the dose does not seem to be clinically important.

The most commonly used and effective statins are simvastatin (which can be bought over the counter), pravastatin and atorvastatin but new ones are coming on stream. Rosuvastatin is one of the newer statins.

Effects of statins:
- reduce LDL cholesterol by 30%
- reduce triglycerides by 20%
- reduce major coronary events by 30%
- reduce cardiac mortality
- reduce coronary procedures (angioplasty and bypass)
- reduce stroke
- reduce total mortality.

Use of statins in primary prevention of cardiovascular disease

Statins should be prescribed to patients, including the elderly, who are at risk of cardiovascular disease. This can be estimated using risk-prediction charts. Patients whose risk is greater than 15% should be prescribed a statin. The limitations of risk-prevention charts are that they do not take into account family history and other emerging risk factors. Dyslipidaemia is not the sole requirement for statins because of their other beneficial effects. Currently, statins are recommended if the total serum cholesterol is ≥5 mmol/l or the estimated 10-year risk of a cardiovascular event is greater than 30%.

Use of statins in secondary prevention of cardiovascular disease

Patients with coronary heart disease, cerebrovascular disease or peripheral artery disease should be prescribed a statin. Statins reduce the risk of non-haemorrhagic stroke when used for secondary prevention in coronary heart disease.

> Statins reduce coronary and cardiovascular events in patients even if the cholesterol level is normal.

Highest dose statins for patients with vascular disease

Each doubling of a statin dose results in a 6% reduction in LDL. Recently, intensive lipid lowering with high-dose statins has been shown to decrease significantly the incidence of myocardial infarction and death, and heart failure independent of recurrent infarction in patients with acute coronary syndromes. High-dose statins also reduce atheroma detected by intravascular ultrasound, possibly by improving the lipid profile (decreasing LDL-cholesterol by 50%, increasing HDL-cholesterol by 15%). High-dose statins also reduced the risk of stroke and coronary events in patients with a recent stroke and no known coronary disease. These results were associated with clinical benefits. This highlights the principle of aggressive lipid lowering in patients with acute myocardial infarction and other acute coronary syndromes, and all forms of vascular disease.

Adverse effects of statins are dose-dependent with 2–3% elevations of liver enzymes, which only rarely result in jaundice. The risk of myopathy increases from 0.2% to 0.6% with statin doses of 80 mg compared with doses of 40 mg (using simvastatin, atorvastatin or pravastatin). These adverse event rates are low, but 80 mg doses have been used in trials for only six months on average and so there is little evidence on their long-term safety profile. It is recommended that patients on highest-dose statins, particularly those who are elderly, frail, or those who have multisystem disorders and those on drugs that may interact, should be monitored more closely, because adverse effects are more likely with higher doses.

Underuse of statins in primary care

GPs and nurse practitioners are becoming increasingly experienced at running lipid clinics, taking blood samples for lipid levels in the surgery and treating patients for both primary and secondary prevention. But for reasons that are unclear, only around half of the total number of patients at risk who should be on statins are being treated. Possible reasons include practitioners' inexperience, lack of awareness of the benefits, over-caution or a concern for thrift. Few clinicians prescribe statins to the recommended maximum dose.

Bile acid sequestrants (e.g. cholestyramine, colestipol)

These have now been largely replaced by statins. Patients find bile acid sequestrants difficult to take because of gastrointestinal pain, wind and constipation. They affect the absorption of other drugs. They:

◇ reduce LDL cholesterol by 15–30%
◇ raise HDL cholesterol by 3–55%
◇ may increase triglycerides and are contraindicated in hypertriglyceridaemia. They reduce the absorption of fat-soluble vitamins and so supplemental vitamins A, D and K are required for patients on long-term treatment.

Bile acid sequestrants reduce major coronary events and reduce cardiac mortality. They are not absorbed and so are the drugs of choice in young women (who may get pregnant) and in children. They are useful in combination with statins and act synergistically to reduce LDL cholesterol.

Nicotinic acid (niacin)

This is used only rarely. It:

✧ lowers LDL cholesterol by 5–25%
✧ lowers triglycerides by 20–50%
✧ raises HDL cholesterol by 15–35%.

The side effects include: flushing, hyperuricaemia, upper gastrointestinal side effects, and liver damage. It is contraindicated in patients with liver disease, diabetes, severe gout and peptic ulcer, and in patients taking warfarin. It reduces major coronary events. Its effects on total mortality are not clear.

Nicotinic acid is available over the counter and is cheap, safe and useful as combination therapy with statins in patients with high triglycerides or persistently raised LDL cholesterol.

Fibrates (e.g. bezafibrate, gemfibrozil, fenofibrate, clofibrate)

Fibrates lower triglyceride levels effectively, elevate HDL and reduce LDL by 18%. They are used mainly to reduce the risk of acute pancreatitis in patients with high triglycerides. Bezafibrate was found to increase HDL cholesterol levels and independently lower cardiac mortality. Clofibrate is rarely used after a trial showed that it was associated with an increase in gastrointestinal tumours and mortality.

Fibrates reduce progression of coronary artery disease and reduce CHD events and non-fatal infarction. They are recommended for high-risk patients with high cholesterol and triglycerides.

Side effects include muscle pain and raised creatine kinase levels particularly in patients with renal impairment, hypothyroidism and when statins are taken in addition.

Torcetrapib

There may be risks associated with increasing HDL cholesterol levels. The torcetrapib trial – torcetrapib is a cholesterylester transfer protein inhibitor – was stopped prematurely due to increased mortality in the torcetrapib and atorvastatin arm of the study in comparison with those using atorvastatin alone.

Antithrombotic therapy

Aspirin is recommended for all patients with vascular disease, and also in diabetics.

Aspirin resistance is believed to be an uncommon problem where, due to arachidonic activity, through a cyclo-oxygenase (COX)-independent mechanism, platelet aggregation occurs causing thrombus formation.

Combined antithrombotic therapy for patients with vascular disease

The combination of aspirin plus clopidogrel was not superior to aspirin alone in reducing cardiovascular death, myocardial infarction and stroke, but did increase the risk of bleeding. However, this combination may be superior to aspirin alone in patients with cerebrovascular disease.

Fish oils

Greenland Eskimos, who eat whale and seal that contain omega-3 polyunsaturated fatty acids (n3-PUFA), have lower levels of total cholesterol, triglycerides, LDL, VLDL but increased HDL and importantly, lower rates of coronary heart disease compared to Danes. In addition, men who eat some fish every week have lower rates of heart disease than those who eat no fish. Not all studies have shown the benefits of eating oily fish but the notion has captured the public imagination and has been widely advocated in the media. The protective role of fish oils in preventing coronary heart disease remains unproven. Fish-oil levels do not correlate with the incidence of myocardial infarction and a large dose of n3-PUFA has no effect on restenosis after coronary angioplasty. However, fish oils in one study did reduce all-cause mortality after myocardial infarction but not by reducing cholesterol. N-3 fatty acids have antiarrhythmic properties and may reduce the risk of sudden death after myocardial infarction.

Patients should be advised to eat fish twice a week rather than fatty foods or dairy products. Even if the evidence for fish as a lipid-lowering or heart-protective food is weak, oily fish would appear to be less likely to increase lipid levels than other foods.

Cholesterol absorption inhibitors

These are new and may be found to be important as adjunctive treatment in resistant cases. They target the exogenous pathway.

Ezetimibe is a new drug which appears to be safe. It is given in a dose of 10 mg a day. It acts by inhibiting the absorption of around 50% of dietary and biliary cholesterol. It does not interfere with the absorption of triglycerides or fat-soluble vitamins. When given alone it reduces LDL cholesterol levels by 20%.

It is not recommended as first-line therapy for either primary or secondary prevention. It may be given as sole therapy to patients with dyslipidaemia who cannot tolerate a statin. It is used as combination therapy with a statin for patients whose cholesterol level remains high despite optimal doses of a statin. Ezetimibe acts synergistically with statins resulting in a reduction in LDL cholesterol of around 40% compared with a reduction of 30% with a statin alone. There is no evidence that ezetimibe combined with simvastatin reduces the progression of atherosclerosis.

Cholesterol ester transfer protein (CTEP) inhibitors

Plasma levels of high-density lipoprotein cholesterol are inversely related to the incidence of coronary heart disease and stroke. The lowering of low-density lipoprotein (LDL) cholesterol with statins reduces the risk of atherosclerotic heart disease by 30%.

Unusual lipid abnormalities

These may need specialist referral. Family members should be evaluated.

Patients with very high LDL levels (>4.9 mmol/l) may need a statin plus a bile acid sequestrant, plus nicotinic acid, but warn the patient about the high risk of side effects.

Very high triglyceride levels (>4.0 mmol/l) are associated with:

⬥ obesity

✧ physical inactivity
✧ cigarette smoking
✧ excess alcohol
✧ type 2 diabetes
✧ chronic renal disease
✧ high carbohydrate intake
✧ steroids.

Secondary causes of hyperlipidaemia

These are listed above and should be treated vigorously.

Uncommon genetic causes of hyperlipidaemia

Familial hypercholesterolaemia

The heterozygote form is inherited as an autosomal dominant and occurs in 1 in 500 people and so most GPs would have at least four patients with this condition.

Patients have very high LDL (>5.0 mmol/l) and total cholesterol levels (>8.0 mmol/l), a family history of hypercholesterolaemia and/or premature coronary artery disease. Look for tendon xanthomata and an arcus (significant in young patients – younger than 50 years). Affected patients need aggressive treatment (often all three classes of lipid-lowering drugs) and specialist referral for diagnosis and monitoring of vascular disease.

Children of affected individuals should be screened at the age of 12 years. Screening family members provides a 50% yield. Affected patients should be referred to a specialist.

The homozygous form is very rare and affected individuals usually die very young from accelerated atherosclerosis.

Which patients with hyperlipidaemia should be referred to a specialist?

✧ Those with resistant hyperlipidaemia.
✧ Those with cardiac symptoms.
✧ Those with side effects to drugs.
✧ Those with other risk factors which are difficult to control.
✧ Non-compliant patients.
✧ Those with possible side effects.
✧ Patients with mixed hyperlipidaemia who may need fibrates and statins.
✧ Patients who want to be referred.

Advice for patients

✧ You can and should do a lot for yourself and we will help you.
✧ Try to change to a healthy, low-fat diet. We will give you advice about this.

- ✧ Losing weight, exercising regularly, avoiding fatty foods and stopping smoking will greatly reduce your risk of a heart attack and stroke.
- ✧ Patients with a high cholesterol or who have had a heart attack, bypass surgery or angioplasty should be taking a statin tablet. Diabetic patients may also need a fibrate.
- ✧ These measures will also improve your chances of a longer and healthier life after a heart attack, coronary artery bypass surgery or angioplasty. You should be taking a statin if you have had any of these conditions.
- ✧ Having a low cholesterol level is very important if you have any cardiovascular risk factor, particularly diabetes or hypertension, or if you are overweight.
- ✧ Make sure your blood pressure is checked regularly and if it is high, take treatment for life.

Answers to questions about clinical cases

1. Ask him if he understands what happened to him; whether he is taking the medication prescribed; what sort of exercise he is doing, and how frequently. Ask him about his diet and if he wants to attend a rehabilitation programme. Explain that he would benefit from a statin and suggest that he tries one.
2. Check her lipids. Unless there are indications for drug intervention, reassure her and give her advice on primary prevention. Offer to see her again if she is anxious.
3. If the patient is having rest pain or symptoms of unstable angina, she should be referred to hospital. Perform a full cardiac evaluation, ECG, lipid profile, full blood count, electrolytes and thyroid function tests and start her on anti-anginal treatment, including aspirin, a statin, a low dose of β-blocker and GTN spray if she is able to use it. Advise her not to over-exert herself for the next few days. If her symptoms do not improve within 48 hours, additional antianginal treatment (e.g. long acting nitrates or nicorandil) can be added.
4. Examine him, consider a statin-induced myopathy, check the CPK, CRP, ESR and liver function tests and if necessary, stop the statin. Consider other causes of muscle pain.
5. Start him on a statin and check his lipids after two months.

FURTHER READING

Department of Health. *National Service Framework for Coronary Heart Disease: modern standards and service models.* London: Department of Health; 2001.

Department of Health. *National Service Framework for Diabetes: standards.* London: Department of Health; 2001.

Handler C, Coghlan G. *Living with Coronary Disease.* London: Springer; 2007.

Sanz J, Moreno PR, Fuster V. The Year in Atherothrombosis. *J Am Coll Cardiol.* 2007; **49:** 1740–9.

Wood D, Wray R, Poulter N, *et al.* JBS:2 Joint British Societies' guidelines on prevention of cardiovascular disease in clinical practice. *Heart.* 2005; **91:** 1–38.

Cholesterol

Afilalo J, Duque G, Steele R, *et al.* Statins for secondary prevention in elderly patients: a hierarchical bayesian meta-analysis. *J Am Coll Cardiol.* 2008; **51**: 37–45.

Cannon CP, Steinberg BA, Murphy SA, Mega JL, Braunwald E. Meta-analysis of cardiovascular outcomes trials comparing intensive versus moderate statin therapy. *J Am Coll Cardiol.* 2006; **48**: 438–45.

Expert Panel on Detection, Evaluation and Treatment of High Blood Cholesterol in Adults. Executive summary of the third report of the National Cholesterol Education Program (NCEP) expert panel on detection, evaluation and treatment of high blood cholesterol in adults (adult treatment panel III). *JAMA.* 2001; **285**: 2486–97.

Hulten E, Jackson JL, Douglas K, George S, Villines TC. The effect of early, intensive statin therapy on acute coronary syndrome. A meta-analysis of randomized controlled trials. *Arch Intern Med.* 2006; **166**: 1814–21.

Neaton J, Wentworth D. (1992) Serum cholesterol, blood pressure, cigarette smoking and death from coronary heart disease. The Multiple Risk Factor Intervention Trial Research Group. *Arch Intern Med.* 1992; **152**: 56–64.

Smoking

Irbarren C, Tekawa IS, Sidney D, Friedman GD. Effect of cigar smoking on the risk of cardiovascular disease, chronic obstructive pulmonary disease, and cancer in men. *N Engl J Med.* 1999; **340**: 1773–80.

Renal function

Adler AI, Stevens RJ, Manley SE, *et al.* Development and progression of nephropathy in type 2 diabetes: the United Kingdom Prospective Diabetes Study (UKPDS 64). *Kidney Int.* 2003; 225–32.

Backer G, Ambrosia E, Borch-Johnson K, *et al.* European guidelines on cardiovascular disease prevention in clinical practice. *Eur J Cardiovasc Prev Rehab.* 2003; **10(Suppl 1)**: S1–S78.

Brantsma AH, Bakker SJ, de Zeeuw D, *et al.* Urinary albumin excretion as a predictor of the development of hypertension in the general population. *J Am Soc Nephrol.* 2006; **17**: 331–5.

Culleton BF, Larson MG, Wilson PW, Evans JC, *et al.* Cardiovascular disease and mortality in a community-based cohort with mild renal insufficiency. *Kidney Int.* 1999; **56**: 2214–9.

Department of Health. *The National Service Framework for Renal Services: Part two: Chronic kidney disease, acute renal failure and end of life care.* London: Department of Health; 2005.

Sattopinto JJ, Fox KAA, Goldberg RJ, *et al.* Creatinine clearance and adverse hospital outcomes in patients with acute coronary syndromes: findings from the global registry of acute coronary events (GRACE). *Heart.* 2003; **89**: 1003–08.

The Royal College of General Practitioners Effective Clinical Practice Unit. *Diabetic renal disease: prevention and early management*; 2002. Available from: www.nice.org.uk?page.aspx?o-39385

Exercise

Sandvik L, Erikssen J, Thaulow E, Mundal R, Rodahl K. Physical fitness as a predictor of mortality among healthy, middle-aged Norwegian men. *N Eng J Med.* 1993; **328**: 533–7.

Obesity

Hubert HB, Feinlib M, McNamara PM, *et al.* Obesity is an independent risk factor for cardiovascular disease: a 26-year follow-up of participants in the Framingham Heart Study. *Circulation.* 1983; **67:** 968–77.

Alcohol

Criqui MH, Ringel BL. Does diet or alcohol explain the French paradox? *Lancet.* 1994; **344:** 1719–23.

Mukamal KJ, Conigrave KM, Mittlemen MA, *et al.* Roles of drinking pattern and type of alcohol consumed in coronary heart disease in men. *N Engl J Med.* 2003; **348:** 109–18.

Thun MJ, Peto R, Lopez AD, *et al.* Alcohol consumption and mortality among middle-aged and elderly US adults. *N Engl J Med.* 1997; **337:** 1705–14.

Lipoprotein (a)

Harjai KJ. Potential new cardiovascular risk factors: left ventricular hypertrophy, homocysteine, lipoprotein (a), triglycerides, oxidative stress, and fibrinogen. *Ann Intern Med.* 1999; **131:** 376–386.

Triglycerides

Avins AL, Neuhaus JM. Do triglycerides provide meaningful information about heart disease risk? *Arch Intern Med.* 2000; **160:** 1937–44.

Fish oils

Kromhout D, Bosschieter EB, de Lezenne-Coulander C. The inverse relationship between fish consumption and 20-year mortality from coronary heart disease. *N Engl J Med.* 1985; **313:** 1205–09.

Vollset SE, Heuch I, Bjelke E. Fish consumption and mortality form coronary heart disease. *N Engl J Med.* 1985; **313:** 820–21.

Hormone replacement treatment

Grodstein F, Stampfer M. The epidemiology of coronary heart disease and estrogen replacement in postmenopausal women. *Prog Cardiovasc Dis.* 1995; **38:** 199–210.

Lokkegaard E, PederseT, Heitmann BL, *et al.* Relation between hormone replacement therapy and ischaemic heart disease in women: prospective observational study. *BMJ.* 2003; **326:** 426–8.

Risks and benefits of estrogen plus progestin in healthy postmenopausal women: principal results from the Women's Health Initiative randomized controlled trial. *JAMA.* 2002; **288:** 321–33.

Homocysteine

Boushey CJ, Beresford SA, Omen CS, Motulsky AG. A quantitative assessment of plasma homocysteine as a risk factor for vascular disease. Probable benefits for increasing folic acid intakes. *JAMA.* 1995; **274:** 1049–57.

Clarke R, Daly L, Robinson K, *et al.* Hyperhomocysteinaemia: An independent risk factor for vascular disease. *N Engl J Med.* 1991; **324:** 1149–55.

Danesh J, Lewington S. Plasma homocysteine and coronary heart disease: systematic review of published epidemiological studies. *J Cardiovasc Risk*. 1998; **5:** 229–32.

Mayer EM, Jacobsen DW, Robinson K. Homocysteine and atherosclerosis. *J Am Coll Cardiol*. 1996; **27:** 517–27.

Family history

Myers RH, Kiely DK, Cupples A, *et al.* Parental history is an independent risk factor for coronary artery disease: the Framingham study. *Am Heart J*. 1990; **120:** 963–9.

Stress

Hemingway H, Marmot M. Psychosocial factors in the aetiology and prognosis of coronary heart disease: systematic review of prospective cohort studies. *BMJ*. 1999; **318:** 1460–7.

Kasterlein JJP, Akdim F, Stroes ESG, *et al.* Simvastatin with or without ezetimibe in familial hypercholesterolaemia. *N Eng J Med*. 2008; **358:** 1431–43.

Kivimäki M, Leino-Arjas P, Luukkonen R, Riihimäki H, *et al.* Work stress and risk of cardiovascular mortality: prospective cohort study of industrial employees. *BMJ*. 2002; **325:** 857–60.

Shen B-J, Avivi YE, Todaro JF, *et al.* Anxiety characteristics independently and prospectively predict myocardial infarction in men. The unique contribution of anxiety among psychologic factors. *J Am Coll Cardiol*. 2008; **51:** 113–19.

Atherosclerosis imaging and screening

SIX

Clinical cases

1. A 43-year-old symptom-free, anxious man with no cardiovascular risk factors is worried about the possibility of having heart disease because his father died, aged 80, apparently from a heart attack. He asks you whether he should have an electron beam computed tomogram (EBCT scan) which is claimed to provide diagnostic information about the presence of heart disease. What advice do you give him?
2. A 68-year-old man who had coronary angioplasty two years ago and who is on aspirin, atenolol and a statin comes to see you for a check-up because he sometimes feels a little breathless but this is not consistently related to exercise. What do you do?
3. A 52-year-old man brings the result of an electron beam computed tomogram calcium score that he had while abroad. It shows a high score. He wants to know if he needs another test. What do you advise him to do?
4. A 64-year-old man, who is at intermediate risk, asks you whether he should have exercise testing or a calcium score done by EBCT scanning. What do you advise him?

Aims of risk stratification and atherosclerosis imaging

Most coronary events – sudden cardiac death, unstable angina or myocardial infarction – are due to rupture of an atheromatous plaque causing less than a 50% stenosis of a coronary artery. Patients with atherosclerosis affecting the carotid, peripheral arteries or aorta are at similar cardiovascular risk to patients with coronary heart disease.

The challenge for clinicians responsible for cardiovascular prevention is to detect coronary atherosclerosis and to predict which individuals are at risk of coronary events. In order to optimise efficacy, safety and cost effectiveness, intensive intervention and drug treatments should be adjusted to the individual's baseline risk.

Patients are categorised into low-, intermediate- and high-risk groups, based on their age, gender and the presence of risk factors. There are several methods to estimate an individual's 10-year cardiovascular risk, which is used to decide whether drugs are appropriate to treat individual risk factors. Patients at low risk are those without vascular disease, who have no major cardiovascular risk factor or family history of premature coronary heart disease. Low-risk individuals have a 10-year cardiovascular risk of less than 10%. Low-risk individuals aged less than 50 years are at very much lower risk than this.

Atherosclerosis imaging, using various techniques, has been used to identify atherosclerosis in arteries with the aim of identifying patients at risk from cardiovascular events who would benefit from prevention measures. The techniques used include carotid artery ultrasound scanning, coronary calcium scanning, cardiovascular magnetic resonance imaging scanning and the ankle-brachial index.

Cost-benefit analysis of atherosclerotic imaging in high- and low-risk individuals

The value and limitations of atherosclerotic imaging are illustrated by comparing the number needed to treat and the cost implications for patients at high and low cardiovascular risk.

High-risk patients

If a treatment reduces the relative risk of cardiovascular death by 25%, then in a high-risk individual with an absolute 10-year risk of 20%, 20 patients will need to be treated for 10 years to prevent one death.

Low-risk individuals

If a low-risk individual has a 1% 10-year risk of cardiovascular death, then 400 individuals must be treated for 10 years to save one life.

Drawbacks to atherosclerotic imaging in low-risk individuals

Before these various techniques are recommended for clinical use, they must provide accurate, reliable, reproducible, cost-effective information which *adds significantly to conventional cardiovascular risk scoring assessments.* At present, there is doubt concerning the widespread use of these techniques in routine clinical practice.

- ✧ Atherosclerotic imaging, including electron beam computed tomography (EBCT) and nuclear perfusion imaging, is not recommended for asymptomatic individuals.
- ✧ The application of atherosclerotic imaging is theoretically best suited to intermediate-risk patients, but before clinicians apply it to these patients, a greater body of supporting evidence is needed to show the incremental benefit of obtaining the information imaging provides. The test must provide significantly more information, over and above conventional risk-factor estimation or other simpler, less dangerous and less expensive non-invasive physiological tests.
- ✧ Because most of what scientists know about the characteristics of vulnerable plaque comes from referred populations in pathology studies, the applicability of the data to clinical screening populations must be demonstrated.
- ✧ Data are needed on the incremental value of new imaging techniques' clinical risk assessment. The methodology used for cardiac imaging needs to be standardised and its reproducibility and variability defined, especially in the case of emerging technologies.
- ✧ Selecting intermediate-risk patients for plaque burden assessment by imaging technology has potential advantages, but more data are needed in low- and high-risk patients.
- ✧ There is a paucity of high-quality outcome and cost-effectiveness data for atherosclerosis imaging and therefore long-term outcome data are needed to develop models of cost effectiveness.

Imaging and other diagnostic tests used for cardiovascular diagnosis and prognosis are most appropriately used in patients at 'intermediate' coronary risk. This can be defined as an annual risk of 0.6% to 2% (10-year risk of 6% to 20%) whereas 'low' risk can be defined as an annual coronary event risk of <0.6% (10-year risk of <6%) and 'high risk' as >2% (10-year risk of 20%).

These tests will not provide further *diagnostic* information in patients with angina or proven coronary artery disease who are at high risk. In *low-risk* individuals, the tests are more likely to provide misleading information and complicate clinical decision-making. At present, atherosclerotic imaging tests are most appropriately used in individuals at *intermediate* risk.

However, there is currently insufficient evidence to support the use of any form of atherosclerotic imaging in individuals in any risk group and their use cannot be recommended. They do not provide additional diagnostic or prognostic information over conventional coronary risk scores combined, where appropriate, with non-invasive stress testing. In addition, there is no evidence that they are cost effective.

Carotid artery ultrasound

This can be used to image carotid artery intima-media thickness, which may be increased in hypertension, and image atherosclerotic plaques. Doppler quantification of carotid artery disease may show obstruction to flow if there is a stenosis of <50%. Intima-media thickness increases with age and this complicates the interpretation of the results. Serial measurements performed by the same person on the same machine may, in the same individual, provide useful information regarding a change in the condition or response to treatment. It cannot be recommended as a screening test.

Coronary calcium calcification by computed tomography scanning

It has been known for many years that the presence of calcium in the walls of coronary arteries seen on X-ray fluoroscopy increases the probability of coronary artery disease although its prognostic significance is unknown. There is no predictable or consistent relationship between the presence of calcium in an artery and the probability of plaque rupture. Plaque rupture is more likely to occur in soft vulnerable plaque than in hard, calcified plaque. The majority of people who have advanced subclinical atherosclerosis are in the low-risk group.

Electron beam computerised axial tomography (EBCT) and multi-detector computed tomography (MDCT) are expensive techniques, not available in NHS hospitals, and used for coronary calcium scanning. They expose the patient to a considerable dosage of ionising radiation equivalent to approximately 15 chest X-rays. The tests provide a 'calcium score'. For men, the probability of having any detectable coronary calcium is roughly equivalent to their age. For women, the probability is 10 to 15 points below their age. Therefore, the calcium score is strongly related to a person's age. The tests are marketed as a component of a risk-factor evaluation but the prognostic value of calcium scoring remains unclear.

There is no evidence that either test to measure coronary artery calcification is helpful as a screening test for coronary artery disease in unselected low-risk patients. In low-risk individuals, coronary artery calcium scoring does not provide incremental predictive value over clinical cardiovascular risk assessment. It has equivalent predictive value as exercise testing and is inferior to magnetic resonance imaging in detecting subclinical atherosclerosis.

In patients at intermediate risk, a high calcium score has similar predictive value as the presence of diabetes or peripheral artery disease. However, the presence of either of these risk factors, even in the absence of symptoms, would be an indication for vigorous risk-factor treatment irrespective of the calcium score. In patients with these conditions, calcium scoring would therefore not influence clinical management and is not recommended.

Recently, calcium screening using EBCT in individuals at intermediate risk was found to provide little additional information over risk estimation using conventional risk factors. In order to get one benefit among people at intermediate risk, 100 women and 60 men would have to be screened. Therefore, even in the intermediate risk group, EBCT scanning is not cost-effective.

Comparison of EBCT scanning with coronary angiography

EBCT scanning does not, in contrast to angiography, provide reliable information on intraluminal (inside the artery) disease but the derived 'score' provides a guide as to whether the individual may have vascular disease.

Compared with coronary angiography, EBCT scanning has a sensitivity of 80% and a very low specificity of 40% (less useful than flipping a coin in excluding coronary artery disease and therefore of particular concern in low-risk individuals). The published literature shows that it has an exceedingly high false-positive rate. The clinical and economic implications of false-positive test results in anxious patients are considerable.

Pitfalls in coronary calcium scoring

Around 50% of scans detect unexpected cardiac findings which, when investigated, are almost always of negligible clinical importance. These usually unnecessary and potentially dangerous tests induce severe anxiety in low-risk or asymptomatic patients.

The proposed rationale for its use is that it can 'quantify' atheromatous plaque. Patients with unstable angina may have a high score but this test would add little to either the diagnosis or the prognosis in this high-risk group and the calcium score is irrelevant to the management. The score is usually low in patients at low risk; for example, in young people who do not have arterial wall calcification.

Young patients with acute coronary syndromes usually do not have hard calcific coronary artery stenoses but rather inflamed, ulcerated plaques and thrombus. An EBCT scan can be misleading in this young or middle-aged group (false negatives). Similarly, elderly people in whom coronary artery calcification is expected may have no intraluminal disease and this results in a high-false positive rate.

The interobserver variability of around 24% and the major variability (50%) in the calcium score reported by the same observer in the same patient scanned on two consecutive days raise important issues in the applicability of this new imaging modality, particularly in those patients in whom it is advocated as a method to monitor response to lipid-lowering treatment.

The test provides no useful clinical information to monitor vascular disease or to guide and monitor treatment in either high- or low-risk patients. It cannot be recommended in asymptomatic patients or as a screening test for selecting asymptomatic patients for invasive investigations. Recommending that asymptomatic patients should adopt a healthy lifestyle and the indications for treating hyperlipidaemia, hypertension or diabetes or to stop smoking, would not be affected by the results of a calcium score.

The results of coronary calcium scoring have been derived mainly from Caucasian men and so should be applied with caution to Caucasian women and people from other ethnic groups.

Much more information is required in individuals with intermediate cardiovascular risk before coronary calcium scoring is recommended. At present, exercise testing remains the test of first choice in patients at intermediate risk. Both exercise testing and stress echocardiography are easily performed, widely available, cheap and safe techniques that can be performed in an outpatient clinic or a doctor's office. Neither test produces radiation.

EBCT scanning may be indicated in the rare case of a patient at intermediate coronary risk (that is, 10–20% 10-year risk) in whom other non-invasive tests are contraindicated or the results cannot be interpreted. Otherwise it is a costly waste of resources.

A thorough clinical assessment incorporating a risk-assessment analysis with simple blood tests and judicious use of exercise testing will suffice for practically all patients. EBCT scanning is not recommended in either high- or low-risk individuals. It has a very limited role in patients at intermediate risk.

Cardiac magnetic resonance imaging (CMR)

Cardiac magnetic resonance imaging has potential for imaging and characterising atherosclerotic plaque and can differentiate different plaque components – fibrous cap, calcium and lipid core. This may provide prognostic information because patients with lipid-rich, unstable, inflamed plaques may be at particularly high risk from coronary events. Carotid arteries are easier to image than the aorta or coronary arteries. Cardiac magnetic resonance imaging can detect silent myocardial scarring and this might prove to be a useful predictor of cardiovascular mortality. Cardiac MR is not widely available and there are no large-scale studies concerning its prognostic value. It is comparatively reproducible and accurate.

Multicontrast, high-resolution magnetic resonance imaging has been used to evaluate the prognostic features of plaque in carotid arteries. Several plaque features (intraplaque haemorrhage, large necrotic core, maximum wall thickness and a thin or ruptured fibrous cap) were found to be strong predictors of subsequent ipsilateral stroke.

Ankle brachial index (ABI)

This is the ratio of the systolic blood pressure at the ankle divided by the systolic blood pressure in the arm. When a stenosis in a peripheral artery reaches a critical level, a decrease occurs in effective perfusion pressure distal to the stenosis and this is roughly equal to the severity of the occlusive disease.

The test is painless, simple to perform and is used in vascular clinics. It detects advanced peripheral artery disease but does not detect early plaque formation. An abnormal ABI is a value less or equal to 0.9 and this has a sensitivity of about 90% and a specificity of about 98%. It can detect subclinical disease and 40% of patients with abnormal ABI results are symptom free.

It is fairly reproducible but not sufficiently so to recommend its use for serial testing but may be used for population screening. It provides incremental predictive information over clinical risk assessment. Its clinical impact is limited by the low prevalence of abnormal test results in individuals younger than 60 years of age. However, it has been shown to be a useful tool to predict future cardiovascular events in the general population after adjustment for potential confounders.

Invasive imaging of atherosclerosis

Intravascular ultrasound (IVUS) is a powerful tool which images atheroma in the coronary arteries. It is performed in only a few UK centres but more widely in Europe and the USA. An ultrasound probe is inserted into coronary arteries in a similar manner as a guidewire and a balloon catheter for coronary angioplasty.

IVUS is used in the evaluation of patients before and after angioplasty and medical treatments for angina. It provides insights into the mechanisms and consequences of myocardial infarction and antiatherosclerotic treatments.

Screening for coronary heart disease in symptom-free individuals
Exercise testing

The main indication for exercise testing is in the assessment of reversible ischaemia in individuals at intermediate risk.

Exercise testing in symptom-free patients with a low pretest probability of coronary heart disease is of limited diagnostic value. In common with other non-invasive tests of ischaemia, it should be performed only after a careful consideration of the pretest likelihood of coronary artery disease in the individual. A 'positive' test result in an individual at low risk is likely to be a 'false-positive' result and must be interpreted with caution with knowledge of the patient's clinical state. A 'negative' test result in a high-risk patient is likely to be a 'false-negative' result and should not affect the need to withhold long-term preventative treatment. However, the absence of ischaemia in a low-risk individual would virtually exclude coronary heart disease and this can be very reassuring and has a therapeutic value.

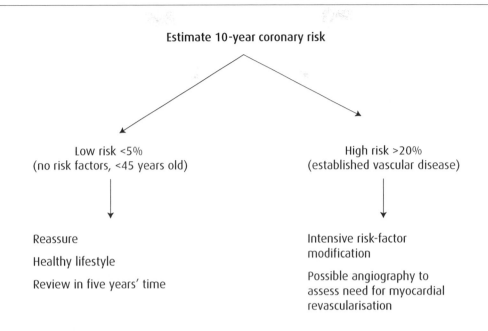

FIGURE 6.1 Screening asymptomatic individuals for coronary artery disease

Advice for patients

✧ At present, the most widely accepted and reliable method of assessing your risk of having heart disease – furring up of your heart arteries – is using a clinical risk-assessment programme. This incorporates a number of factors and we can then get an idea of your risk. You will need to have a clinical examination to measure your blood pressure, and a blood test to check your sugar (glucose) and cholesterol levels.

✧ If you have angina or claudication, or have had a heart attack or angioplasty or heart bypass surgery, or have a problem in the blood supply to your brain, you have furring up in at least one of the arteries in your body. This means you are at high risk and should do everything you can to reduce your risk. We can help you with this.

✧ You are more likely to have furring up in your arteries, and are more likely to develop furred-up arteries, if you have a risk factor. Examples of risk factors are if you smoke or have smoked recently, have a high blood pressure (more than 140/85 mmHg), are diabetic, have a high cholesterol level, if you are overweight and if you do not exercise regularly.

✧ Doctors can almost always get the necessary information about your risk and the probability of your having furred-up arteries by simple clinical methods and an exercise test or other stress test.

Answers questions about clinical cases

1. EBCT is not recommended for individuals at low risk or at high risk. There is some support for its use in a small number of intermediate-risk individuals. However, conventional clinical assessment, with exercise testing if appropriate, is recommended in this patient. Generally, EBCT scanning is not recommended for screening.

2. Check his blood pressure, examine him for possible causes of breathlessness, check his lipid status, and do haematology biochemical tests. Arrange a chest X-ray and ECG. If all these are satisfactory, arrange an exercise test to look for exercise performance, blood pressure and heart rate response, reason for stopping exercise and ECG changes. If this test is satisfactory and there is no reason to suspect a lung problem, reassure him and ask him to start exercising. Review him in a few weeks' time.

3. He is at high risk based on the calcium score and, like other high-risk patients (for example, those with diabetes), he should have intensive secondary prevention. There is no evidence that further non-invasive testing (nuclear testing) will result in more appropriate selection of treatments. All secondary prevention targets should be aimed for.

4. Coronary artery calcium scoring has not been compared with other non-invasive tests in risk assessment. However, exercise testing and stress echocardiography do not expose patients to radiation and are less expensive than EBCT. Currently, he should be advised to have an exercise stress test.

FURTHER READING

ACC/AHA. Clinical Expert Consensus Document on coronary artery calcium scoring by computed tomography in global cardiovascular risk assessment and in evaluation of patients with chest pain. *J Am Coll Cardiol.* 2007; **49:** 378–402.

Burke AP, Virmani R, Galis Z, *et al.* Task Force # 2 – What is the pathologic basis for new atherosclerosis imaging techniques? *J Am Coll Cardiol.* 2003; **41:** 1874–86.

Daly C, Saravanan P, Fox K. Is calcium the clue? *Eur Heart J.* 2002; **23:** 1562–6.

Detrano RC, Wong ND, Doherty TM, *et al.* Coronary calcium does not accurately predict near-term future coronary events in high-risk adults. *Circulation.* 1999; **99:** 2633–8. (Errata. *Circulation.* 2000; **101:** 697, 1355.)

Greenland P, Gaziano JM, *et al.* Selecting asymptomatic patients for coronary computed tomography or electrocardiographic exercise testing. *N Engl J Med.* 2003; **349:** 465–73.

Handler C, Coghlan G. *Living with Coronary Disease.* London: Springer; 2007. pp. 236–7.

Mark DB, Shaw LJ, Lauer MS, *et al.* Task Force # 5 – Is atherosclerosis imaging cost effective? *J Am Coll Cardiol.* 2003; **41:** 1906–17.

O'Hare AM, Katz R, Shlipak MG, Cushman M, Newman AB. Mortality and cardiovascular risk across the ankle-arm index spectrum: results from the Cardiovascular Health Study. *Circulation.* 2006; **113:** 388–93.

Pasternak RC, Abrams J, Greenland P, *et al.* Task Force # 1 – Identification of coronary heart disease risk: is there a detection gap? *J Am Coll Cardiol.* 2003; **41:** 1863–74.

Redberg RF, Vogel RA, Criqui MH, *et al.* Task Force # 3 – What is the spectrum of current and emerging techniques for the non-invasive measurement of atherosclerosis? *J Am Coll Cardiol.* 2003; **41:** 1886–98.

Taylor AJ, Merz CNB, Udelson JE. Executive summary – Can atherosclerosis imaging techniques improve the detection of patients at risk for ischaemic heart disease? *J Am Coll Cardiol.* 2003; **41**: 1860–2.

Wilson PWF, Smith SC, Blumenthal RS, *et al.* Task Force # 4 – How do we select patients for atherosclerosis imaging? *J Am Coll Cardiol.* 2003; **41**: 1898–1906.

Obesity and diet

SEVEN

Clinical cases

1. A 48-year-old woman, who is moderately overweight and who finds it difficult to maintain an optimum weight, asks you whether she should go on to the Atkins diet. What do you advise her?
2. A 60-year-old man who is overweight, inactive and drinks one bottle of red wine per day, comes to see you two weeks after leaving hospital for management of unstable angina. He believes that red wine prevented him from having a heart attack and wants you to confirm this. What do you tell him?
3. A 36-year-old diabetic man with a family history of premature coronary heart disease has succeeded in giving up smoking but is now overweight and wants help. How do you help him?
4. A 28-year-old woman who is obese brings her obese 11-year-old daughter to see you because the daughter is being bullied at school because she is fat. What advice do you give?
5. A 60-year-old woman with severe obesity and hypertension manages to lose a considerable amount of weight by going on to a strict, extreme regime of slimming drinks. Over the course of another few months, she puts on nearly all the weight she has lost. Her blood pressure remains high. She would like to lose weight and understands the health implications of obesity but does not want to use the slimming drinks again. What do you advise her to do?
6. A 64-year-old woman who has struggled with her weight all her life, and who has been on several different diets for over 30 years, asks you whether she should try a WeightWatchers™ programme or diet tablets. What do you advise her?

Public health issues

More than 60% of the UK adult population are either overweight or obese. The increasing prevalence of obesity is a major public health issue. It is a reversible cause of reduced life expectancy (30 000 deaths per year), loss of income and tax from sickness absence (18 million days of work are taken off for sickness each year); the associated conditions are a major drain on public health and welfare resources. It is estimated to cost the economy in England £3.7 billion per year. This figure has increased due to the availability of medical and surgical treatments, and the inclusion of the costs of associated conditions.

The implications of obesity are now widely debated and, in common with tobacco and alcohol, considered important public health issues and subjects for Government regulation.

Obesity is likely to become a more important cause of premature death than smoking.

An effective public health policy is required to attack the main causes of obesity. This policy might be similar to that for smoking cessation. Initiatives that have been suggested in the USA include:

✧ widespread public education for all age groups
✧ warning labels and menu information in all restaurants
✧ simple warning labels on food products
✧ legislation for tax incentives for industry to promote health at work
✧ taxation of fatty and other unhealthy food
✧ making it attractive, easy and inexpensive for people of all ages to do daily exercise.

Obesity is associated with diabetes, hypertension, dyslipidaemia, physical inactivity and depression. These conditions significantly increase the risk of cardiovascular death.

TABLE 7.1 Relative risk of other diseases in obese adults

DISEASE	RELATIVE RISK	
	Women	Men
Type 2 diabetes	13	5
Hypertension	4	3
Heart attack	3	2
Colon cancer	3	3
Angina	2	2
Gall bladder disease	2	2
Ovarian cancer	2	–
Osteoarthritis	1	2
Stroke	1	1

(Source: Adapted from National Audit Office data; 2001)

> Type 2 diabetes, hypertension, dyslipidaemia, breathlessness (in the absence of other causes), fatigue and depression (particularly in children who may experience psychosocial problems), may resolve completely in overweight or obese adults as a result of weight loss combined with regular exercise and a healthy diet.

Role of the primary care team in the prevention and management of obesity

Primary care is the focal point for the management of obesity and its complications. Some primary care units have dedicated staff to run obesity and diet clinics.

The management of obesity is rewarding but hard work for primary care clinicians, necessitating enthusiasm, commitment, knowledge of the main pathological process of energy imbalance as the cause of obesity, cardiovascular risk factors and their importance and management, sensitivity, and interpersonal skills. Effective treatment of this increasingly common medical condition requires skill, and a good understanding of the medical, social and psychological profile of the patient.

> Achieving an ideal weight is probably the single most important goal in cardio-vascular prevention. This is because of the risk factors associated with obesity.
>
> Patients will only change their eating habits and increase their exercise if they want to. They need to understand the benefits of weight loss and maintaining their optimum weight.

Patients who remain obese despite a serious trial of calorie restriction and exercise may benefit from drug therapy. Occasionally, surgery and other procedures for obesity (bariatric surgery) may be considered. There are risks with all these interventions and these risks have to be understood and balanced against the risks of severe obesity in the individual patient. These options should be discussed with patients only after all other low-risk methods have been adequately tried.

Primary care clinicians may wish to provide weight management and maintenance services with lay dieting groups in the community (for example, WeightWatchers™), Primary Care Trusts, and hospital specialists. The cost-effectiveness of these services is not known. The costs would be in personnel and their time, but it is likely that among a sizeable community, the long-term cost savings in healthcare would be substantial.

Health promotion and healthy eating

The prevalence of obesity is increasing in children. Nearly 20% of boys and girls in the UK are obese and this percentage has doubled in the last 10 years. Obese children are more likely than slim children to have at least one obese parent. Although most people who are obese were slim as children, obese children often become obese adults. Children and adults who are not obese or even overweight should also be educated about maintaining a healthy weight as part of a primary care health promotion programme. Taking a dietary history does not take long and it is a useful way to help patients think about what they eat and how this can be improved. Most patients welcome this and are grateful to clinicians for taking an interest in this part of their lives. Patients may not consider diet to be a medical problem or something to discuss with a doctor or nurse.

> Obese children often become obese adults. Adults and children should be educated about food and calories so that they understand what they can do to improve their health and reduce their cardiovascular risk.

Parents have to take responsibility for training and educating their children about sensible, healthy eating and the dangers of obesity. Parents have to educate by example.

Without this leadership, it is highly likely that children will develop unhealthy eating habits and are likely to become overweight or obese.

Periods during life when people may become overweight:
✧ prenatal period
✧ rapid growth during infancy
✧ rapid growth in childhood
✧ adolescence and new eating habits, particularly in girls
✧ young adulthood (late teens for females, 20s and 30s in males)
✧ pregnancy
✧ menopause
✧ middle age in men and women (middle-age spread).

Diagnosing obesity

Obesity is an important and increasingly common medical condition which increases medical and cardiovascular risk. It is an excess of body fat and is measured using the body mass index (BMI) or waist circumference.

Most of us know if we are overweight. Obese patients understand that they have a problem but many feel helpless and unable to help themselves, and are resigned to being obese, which they may perceive as a permanent affliction or disability.

TABLE 7.2 Definitions of excess body weight related to body mass index and waist circumference

CATEGORY	BMI (KG/M²)	WAIST CIRCUMFERENCE IN CMS (2.5 CM = 1 INCH)
Normal	18–24	<65 women; <87.5 men
Overweight	25–29	>65 women; >87.5 men
Obese	>30	>87.5 women; >100 men

Methods of measuring obesity

A good set of weighing scales and a height ruler are used to record weight and body mass index (BMI) calculated as weight (in kg) divided by height (in m²). Special scales are necessary for obese patients. It is preferable that people are weighed wearing light clothes, in bare feet, fasting, and after they have emptied their bladder.

Body mass index has been the preferred index to measure obesity and minimises the effect of height on body weight. An increased BMI increases the risk of death from a cardiac cause.

Abdominal obesity is recognised as a major risk factor for cardiovascular disease. Waist circumference, skin fold thickness, and waist : hip ratio appear to be more strongly associated with cardiovascular events and death than BMI. This may be due to excess visceral adipose tissue which promotes insulin resistance, dyslipidaemia and hypertension. Waist : hip ratio may be superior to waist circumference as a predictor of cardiovascular risk because it incorporates a measurement of hip circumference which is inversely associated with insulin resistance, and other biochemical abnormalities underlying the metabolic syndrome. Both should be measured and recorded in patients' records although it is easier to measure waist circumference because patients do not need to disrobe. The cut-off values of these measurements determining cardiovascular risk are not validated.

The waist circumference in men should be less than 87 cm and in women less than 65 cm. Waist sizes greater than 100 cm for men, and 88 cm for women indicate a high risk of type 2 diabetes, coronary heart disease and hypertension, and metabolic syndrome.

> Obesity is a disease causing morbidity and mortality for which the patient has responsibility, and the ability to control.

Prevalence and causes of obesity

The prevalence of obesity is increasing worldwide. Obesity is common in all age groups in the UK and the USA, and is becoming more common, particularly in children. In the USA, 18% of adolescents are overweight. This is due both to the popularity and low cost of 'fast food' (cheap food, containing a high proportion of fat, salt and sugar), and children leading a more sedentary life, doing less sport both in and out of school. Adults in the UK are also working long hours and they have less time for regular exercise and a balanced diet. Many young adults may not eat regular meals, and may go to the pub after work with friends and colleagues, rather than go home to prepare a nutritious meal.

The UK population is aware that exercise is an important part of a healthy lifestyle but generally remains inactive and has an unhealthy diet.

Changing these important causes of obesity requires a major long-term change in a person's lifestyle. Only the person involved is able to make a long-term change to their lifestyle.

Obesity and food choices

Governments recognise the economic and health risks of obesity, and food manufacturers now have a responsibility to list food constituents on food packaging. The choice of food, and the wide availability of a variety of snacks, confectionery, ready prepared meals, and drinks, has increased over the last 30 years. These foods are generally high in calories. To most people, however, food labels mean little because they do not understand how much fat, carbohydrate, protein and energy they should have during a day. Adding up the cost of their shopping is difficult enough and trying to calculate the calorific content of the food would, for most people, be impractical. Most people do not understand how many grams of fat, protein and carbohydrate are desirable or safe. Shopping habits are difficult to change and are formulated by a complex mix of upbringing, taste, budget, convenience, mood or impulse at the time of purchase, and the requests of family and others.

Although 'organic' foods have become quite popular over the last few years, the quality of food does not appear to be the overriding priority of most people in the UK. There is little or no evidence that 'organic' foods are healthier, or are less likely to cause cancer or any other medical problem. However, the reasons that people buy certain foods are not well understood. It is believed that advertising by food manufacturers plays an important role.

The role of Government and economic considerations

Although there is legislation banning smoking in public places, and the wearing of seat belts in motor vehicle, there is currently no UK legislation aimed at improving nutrition and physical activity among children and adults. The powers and duties of Government in regulating private behaviour in order to promote public health have to be defined and balanced against civil liberties. There are also significant pressures from food producers and retailers. It is very unlikely that the restrictions placed on smokers would be applied to the obese.

Evidence that obesity is a significant independent health risk has been established only recently.

Health pressure groups have proposed a number of initiatives for Government-driven and Government-endorsed public health measures. These include the following:

✧ a national obesity agency
✧ an obesity 'black spot' map of the UK
✧ an obesity curriculum and training for healthcare professionals
✧ obesity and food education for school children
✧ increase formal exercise for children in and out of school hours
✧ fat content labelling on foods
✧ encouragement to cycle with cycle lanes on roads and exercise facilities in housing complexes
✧ a ban on the advertising of unhealthy, high-calorie foods
✧ support and funding of obesity surgery for people with a BMI >40
✧ taxing of processed foods with a high calorie content.

Arguments against legislation

Arguments against legislation to curb obesity include civil rights-orientated consumer issues, including 'paternalistic intervention into lifestyle choices', and 'enfeebling of personal responsibility'. Food is considered essential for health rather than a dangerous drug and therefore people should be able to buy whatever they choose. The argument is that government should concern itself with more important public service matters rather than intrude into the personal choices of the public.

Arguments for legislation

Arguments for legislation to curb obesity include the following. Some foods, for example, confectionery and chocolate, are not nutritious and have no health benefits. People buy what they like to eat, what is available and affordable. If calorie-dense foods become less available, more expensive and less well advertised, then people would buy less. Healthy food, fruit and vegetables are not necessarily more expensive than processed foods.

The food industry uses advertising to increase sales. Profit not health promotion, is the nature of the business. A ban on advertising of unhealthy foods will reduce sales. Conversely, advertising of healthy foods would increase sales. However, the food industry does not manufacture fresh food and eating more healthy fresh food, which is not necessarily more expensive than processed food, would displace processed foods from supermarket trolleys and would not be in the industry's interests.

Obesity is a consequence of a voluntary behavioural problem. Food is essential for life and, although in excess it carries health risks to the individual and resource implications for society, it does not carry the same stigma as tobacco, alcohol, or other addictive substances. If it did, then there would be less moral and practical objection to the causes of obesity. Currently, the consumption of excess calorie-dense food is not considered a danger but the cause of an individual's unfortunate cosmetic problem and solely the business of the person concerned. Interference by Government in what or how much an individual wants to eat or drink is frowned upon, as such consumption is seen as a matter for the individual. It has been suggested that obesity may be more common in people in lower socio-economic classes, although this is not clear. Obesity in children and adults occurs in all socio-economic classes. There are practical and moral issues in legislating against unhealthy food or preventing people from eating it.

Possible approaches to reducing obesity through public health initiatives

This is most effectively done through education of families and children at home and in schools. There should also be evidence in large populations that interventions to reduce obesity allow people to live a longer and healthier life. These were the steps leading to the ban on tobacco advertising and banning of smoking in public places.

There has been recent television publicity about the poor quality of school meals and this has had an impact in making school meal providers conscious and careful of their duties in providing children with nutritionally safe food. Schools have been banned from providing sugar-sweetened drinks in vending machines. So far, in the UK, there have not been bans on advertising of specific foods. There are requirements for food labelling. Higher taxation of junk foods, making them more expensive, would probably reduce consumption but this has not been evaluated. In the same way as children are taught about the dangers of smoking and taking drugs, nutrition lessons at schools, if well presented, are likely to be helpful in educating children about food and the dangers of obesity. The NHS provides treatment and help for patients who drink excessive alcohol, and for those who smoke, as well as for those who are obese. Not to do so could be considered discriminatory.

Health risks of obesity

- ✧ Hypertension.
- ✧ Dyslipidaemia.
- ✧ Diabetes.
- ✧ Cardiovascular disease.
- ✧ Lung disease.

❖ Pancreatitis.
❖ Fatty liver.
❖ Gall bladder disease.
❖ Musculoskeletal problems, osteoarthritis in weight-bearing joints, low back pain.
❖ Skin disorders.
❖ Gout.
❖ Tiredness, snoring and poor-quality sleep (sleep apnoea), lack of energy, breathlessness.
❖ Psychological distress, low self-esteem, depression.
❖ Menstrual disorders, infertility, miscarriage, foetal abnormalities, pregnancy-induced hypertension, pre-eclampsia, gestational diabetes, venous thromboembolism, haemorrhage, infection, foetal distress, increased foetal risk of spina bifida, heart defect.
❖ Erectile dysfunction.

Obesity, cardiovascular disease and heart failure

Obese people are predisposed to diabetes, hypertension, left ventricular hypertrophy, stroke, heart failure and heart attack. Overweight children may become overweight adults because dietary and lifestyle habits established in childhood are difficult to change. Most elderly people are slim probably because obese people die before reaching old age. The risks of obesity are more potent in Afro-Caribbean people.

Obesity and cardiac death

Obesity increases the risk of cardiac death. The mechanism may be due to premature coronary artery disease, heart failure and sudden death due to arrhythmia related to left ventricular dilatation and hypertrophy. Ventricular ectopic beats, possibly leading to more serious ventricular arrhythmias, are more common in hypertrophic hearts. The hypertrophy is not concentric as in hypertension, but eccentric, and so the cardiac enlargement in obesity may not simply reflect associated hypertensive heart disease. Obesity results in an increase in blood volume and cardiac output. There are abnormalities in haemodynamics with increased cardiac work during exercise.

Obesity and diabetes

Most type 2 diabetics are overweight or obese and have a BMI of at least 27 kg/m². Waist measurement is probably a better indicator of type 2 diabetes. Increased weight is the major cause of diabetes in young people. Blood sugar levels often reduce to normal when obese people lose weight to attain their optimal weight.

Obesity and hypertension

Hypertension increases as BMI increases and. It may be possible to stop antihypertensive medication in obese people with hypertension after they have lost weight and exercise regularly. It may also be possible to reduce the number of antihypertensive drugs prescribed in obese hypertensives after they have lost weight.

Obesity and dyslipidaemia

Total cholesterol, LDL cholesterol and triglyceride levels are higher, and HDL cholesterol levels are lower in obese individuals. Weight loss, with a low-fat diet combined with exercise, reduces the levels of unfavourable lipids.

Obesity and complications during pregnancy

The risks of developing hypertension or pre-eclampsia are two to three times higher in overweight and obese women compared to women with a normal body mass index. Blood pressure in obese people should be measured using a large cuff.

Gestational diabetes is four times more likely to occur in overweight women and increases the risk by several times of developing diabetes after pregnancy. Weight loss and dietary advice should be given during and after pregnancy and women should be monitored and managed actively in primary care to reduce their risk of developing diabetes.

Obesity increases the risk of thromboembolism and pulmonary emboli, which are the major cause of maternal death in the UK. Obesity trebles the risk of thrombosis. Factor VIII and factor IX levels are higher in obesity.

Children born to obese mothers are believed to be at higher cardiovascular risk. The cause of this observation is not known but it may be due to poor foetal nutrition, or abnormalities in insulin production.

Erectile dysfunction

Erectile dysfunction occurs in around 50% of men aged 40–70 years and is more common in obese men, perhaps because of the metabolic syndrome. Diet, weight loss and daily exercise to reduce obesity and its complications, combined with phosphodiesterase-5 inhibitors, are effective treatment in most people.

Genetics of obesity

The reasons that some people like to eat more in one meal than others remain unclear. Appetite is dependent on hormonal signals from adipose tissue providing feedback to the hypothalamus. A genetic link to childhood obesity has been reported. Melanocyte-stimulating hormone produced in the hypothalamus stimulates the melanocortin 4 receptor (MC4R), which may account for 6% of cases of obesity by influencing the appetite and eating behaviour in affected people.

Obesity as a cardiovascular risk factor

> Obesity is now considered to be as important an independent risk factor for cardio-vascular disease and heart failure as are diabetes, hypertension and smoking. Obesity is also a risk factor for stroke.

Obesity increases the risk of coronary heart disease by 40%. Therefore, obesity as an isolated condition (although it would be unusual for an obese patient to have no other risk factor) increases the risk of stroke and myocardial infarction. It is, however, commonly associated with type 2 diabetes mellitus, hypercholesterolaemia, and hypertension. These conditions are more resistant to treatment in obese patients. They act synergistically as cardiovascular risk factors so that patients with two or more of these conditions are at particularly high risk from cardiac events.

Obese survivors of myocardial infarction have a higher subsequent cardiac risk (i.e. are more likely to have another possibly fatal infarct or develop angina or heart failure) compared to thin patients.

Childhood obesity

Obesity is more common in children today than a generation ago and this is probably due to increased calorie intake and reduced physical activity. The fast-food and snack culture, displacing lower-calorie family meals, together with the near disappearance of organised, compulsory sports at school, are believed to be major factors in this important problem, which predisposes overweight and obese children to becoming overweight and obese adults.

Increasing physical activity alone, without reducing calorie intake, has little effect on weight. Childhood obesity is most likely to be effectively tackled by changing children's eating habits and tastes from a young age until adulthood and beyond. The habit and pleasure of regular effective exercise should be instilled in children by parents, older siblings, teachers and popular youth role models.

> The foundations of a child's attitude to health, diet, exercise, work, relationships, religion and most other aspects of life are more likely to be impressively and effectively seeded at home by their parents rather than from a teacher at school.

The metabolic syndrome

There are six slightly different definitions of metabolic syndrome (proposed by different bodies), which affects around 25% of the population. All include the same core criteria but use different cut-off levels. Insulin resistance and a large waist circumference are the two key characteristics.

At least three of the following features are required for the diagnosis:

- ◇ visceral obesity >102 cm (>40 inches) for men; >88 cm (>35 inches) for women
- ◇ glucose intolerance that contributes to insulin resistance – the core of the problem – and a heightened risk of diabetes, thrombosis and cardiovascular disease; fasting glucose >6.1 mmol/l
- ◇ atherogenic dyslipidaemia (low levels of high-density lipoprotein cholesterol and elevated levels of total cholesterol, low-density lipoprotein cholesterol and triglycerides) HDL <1.0 mmol/l; triglycerides >1.7 mmol/l

✧   elevated C-reactive protein levels
✧   hypertension >130/85 mmHg.

The world prevalence of metabolic syndrome is increasing due to lifestyle changes. This will increase the incidence and prevalence of coronary heart disease. Metabolic syndrome is believed to have a genetic basis in 25% of patients.

Visceral obesity causes insulin resistance and hyperglycaemia, and dyslipidaemia. These changes lead to inflammatory changes in the arterial wall, vessel injury, atherosclerosis and a prothrombotic state.

The predictive value of metabolic syndrome is not established, but the association of several characteristics emphasises the important cardiovascular risk factors associated with obesity and the fact that these risk factors may disappear with significant weight loss. Cardiovascular risk should not be estimated using a diagnosis of metabolic syndrome alone, but by using all validated cardiovascular risk factors (for example, age, LDL cholesterol level, smoking, blood pressure). A diagnosis of metabolic syndrome is a more powerful predictor of cardiovascular events in young people (aged less than 50 years) than in older patients.

Management of metabolic syndrome

Patient education is vital. Patients should be told that obesity is the central component of the problem. Significant weight loss and daily exercise may be sufficient to lower the blood pressure, improve dyslipidaemia and high blood sugar, and make patients feel better. A low-fat, low-carbohydrate diet is fundamental. Cardiovascular risk prediction charts underestimate the 10-year cardiovascular risk in patients with metabolic syndrome and so lower thresholds for starting a statin are reasonable.

Drugs for metabolic syndrome

Metformin and thiazolidenediones (glitazones) are used to correct hyperglycaemia.

Metformin is the only available biguanide. It decreases gluconeogenesis and increases peripheral utilisation of glucose. It works only if there is some residual functioning insulin. It is the drug of first choice in overweight patients. It should not be used in patients with renal impairment and should be stopped a day before patients have angiography or a general anaesthetic.

The thiazolidinediones lower glucose levels by reducing peripheral insulin resistance. Statins and fibrates are used to correct the dyslipidaemia.

Obesity and heart failure

The greater the body mass index, the greater the risk of heart failure. The risk of heart failure in obese people is twice as high compared with the risk for those with a normal body mass index. This risk appears to be independent of other risk factors associated with obesity.

> The symptoms of obesity are similar to those of heart failure (breathlessness, orthopnoea, and oedema) and this makes it difficult to diagnose heart failure in obese people.

Obesity and sleep apnoea syndrome

Obese people often have sleep apnoea and hypoventilation. Sleep apnoea is an important trigger of pulmonary hypertension and has been implicated in the development of coronary heart disease. Affected patients are characteristically obese, fall asleep in the middle of the day and snore loudly because of upper airways obstruction. They have prolonged episodes of apnoea, which frightens their family. Sleep apnoea responds to weight loss. Occasionally, surgery to the upper airways may be necessary.

Benefits of weight loss

A 10% weight loss in obese people results in a:
❖ 20% fall in all-cause mortality
❖ 30% fall in diabetes-associated death
❖ 40% decrease in obesity-related death
❖ fall of 10% in total cholesterol
❖ 15% fall in LDL cholesterol
❖ 30% fall in triglycerides
❖ 8% increase in HDL cholesterol
❖ fall of 10 mmHg in systolic and diastolic blood pressure in hypertensive patients
❖ fall of 50% in fasting glucose in newly diagnosed patients with type 2 diabetes.

Overweight patients with heart conditions, particularly hypertension, type 2 diabetes and hypercholesterolaemia, should be encouraged to lose weight and exercise regularly.

Hypertension may resolve after significant weight loss and so patients with suspected hypertension may not need to start medication or be able to stop their tablets.

Type 2 diabetes may be controlled by diet and weight loss alone.

A low-fat diet and exercise may make statin treatment unnecessary in patients with *mild hyperlipidaemia*.

Patients should also be told that *weight loss improves survival after heart attacks and lowers the risk of stroke*.

Usually, *a weight loss of 4 kg allows antihypertensive medication to be reduced* possibly by reducing the sensitivity of blood pressure to sodium.

Most overweight patients with angina or heart failure improve symptomatically after they lose weight. Because there have not been any randomised controlled trials of weight reduction in obese patients with coronary artery disease, it is not clear whether weight loss alone reduces the risk of cardiac events in secondary prevention. Even in the absence of 'evidence' from a controlled trial, overweight coronary patients should be helped and encouraged to lose weight because losing weight reduces cardiovascular risk.

Benefits of a low-fat diet and lowering cholesterol levels

Reducing fat intake and lowering total and LDL-cholesterol levels reduce the risk of death and cardiovascular events in primary prevention. In patients with coronary artery disease, this benefit occurs even in patients with a normal cholesterol level. Statins are prescribed as part of secondary prevention for patients with any type of atheromatous vascular disease, irrespective of the cholesterol level because of their multiple effects. They reduce inflammation in the arterial wall, improve renal function, and reduce thrombosis.

A low-fat diet reduces the frequency and severity of angina and this may be explained by a change in the behaviour or vasoreactivity of coronary arteries, possibly through an action on nitric oxide.

The US National Cholesterol Education Program Population Panel has estimated that adherence to its recommendations would reduce the cholesterol level in the population by 10% with a reduction in the development of atherosclerosis and its effects on the heart and brain arteries. This 10% reduction in the cholesterol level in the population would prevent 30% of all coronary heart disease events. Treating the patients in the top 10% bracket of cholesterol levels with lipid-lowering drugs would reduce the incidence of coronary events by 20%.

Attitudes to and perceptions about diets

Some patients may be very sensitive about their weight and may not want to discuss what they consider a very personal issue. Before giving dietary advice, it is worthwhile asking patients whether they want to lose weight. It should not be assumed that all overweight or obese patients want to lose weight; most do, but do not wish to change to their diet. Others are prepared to diet as long as they can eat and drink what they want. This is the common perception of a 'good' diet.

Some patients may feel that diets and changes in eating habits are for fat people who simply want to improve their appearance. Giving well-intentioned dietary advice to patients who find it offensive or insulting is dispiriting and a waste of time. Most patients with cardiac conditions are, however, pleased to receive advice and expect it when they visit the surgery. Indeed, patients with cardiac conditions may be disappointed if dietary advice is not given.

Most patients are interested to know how their diet affects their heart and their health and would expect to be asked about their fat, sugar, alcohol, and carbohydrate intake in the same way as they would expect to be asked about smoking and alcohol. They may have read or heard about certain additives, minerals or vitamin supplements and may ask their GP or practice nurse about these and whether they should take them.

Patients are now better informed about diet and 'lifestyle' and know that foods with a high fat and sugar content are 'bad' and increase the risk of coronary heart disease. Although patients may find it very difficult to follow the dietary advice offered, they usually like to know how their diet compares with a 'healthy' diet. A detailed dietary history has to be obtained in order for the clinician to understand why the patient is obese or overweight. Most of us underestimate the amount of fat and alcohol we consume.

Patients want a quick, painless 'fix' with significant weight loss that will be noticed by others. Dieting is popular and a constant feature in all quarters of the media. There are several television programmes about obesity and diet and celebrity chefs also provide low-calorie recipes. Cooking and diet books are usually in the 'bestsellers' list. There are many 'wonder' diets but in general they are tried by the desperate and result in frustration and disappointment rather than long-term weight loss.

Patients need to understand that if they eat less food, particularly fat and carbohydrate, and drink less alcohol, they will lose weight, feel better, live longer and probably need fewer tablets. These benefits will be lost if they revert to their 'old habits' of eating and drinking which will inevitably lead to them regaining the weight they worked so hard to lose. The difficulty in losing weight is not the theory but its practice and maintenance!

General principles of a healthy low-fat diet as part of cardiovascular prevention

The patient's usual daily diet, pattern of eating and exercise activities should be recorded. It is helpful for the patient to bring an accurate record of a typical week's food consumed, including snacks.

A wide variety of foods should be eaten. Calorie reduction and avoidance of saturated fat and carbohydrate are the most effective ways to lose weight. Alcohol is fattening and this should be cut out or consumed only in small quantities.

Salt reduction is important, particularly in hypertension. Salt is found in large quantities in ready prepared meals, fast food, and bread.

Fats

Fats are essential in small amounts to carry vitamins A, D, E and K in the blood, to manufacture prostaglandins and cell membranes. They add flavour, texture and aroma to food and promote a feeling of fullness.

Saturated fats and cardiovascular disease

These are lauric, myristic, palmitic and stearic fats. They are hard at room temperature. Foods rich in saturated fat are meat and dairy products, and vegetable oils, e.g. coconut, and palm oil. It has been known for more than 20 years from the landmark Seven Countries Study that there is a direct relationship between the quantity of saturated fat intake and coronary heart disease event rates. Finland, with high levels of saturated fat intake, had the highest coronary heart disease mortality and Japan, with the lowest saturated fat intake, the lowest mortality. Japanese people who migrated to the US developed higher cholesterol levels and a correspondingly higher rate of coronary heart disease events. Britain, particularly Scotland, has – compared with Mediterranean countries – a high incidence of coronary heart disease and the population has a high intake of saturated fat. An explanation for the lower coronary mortality in obese Italians compared with obese Americans is their saturated fat intake. Italians eat more olive oil and pasta, eat less animal fat, and drink more red wine than Americans who consume a diet high in saturated fat including hamburgers and hot dogs.

Trans-fatty acids

These are found in vegetable oils, margarines, shortenings in cakes and biscuits, milk, butter and cheese. They increase cholesterol.

Unsaturated fatty acids

These lower LDL cholesterol when substituted for saturated fat. They are liquid at room temperature.

Polyunsaturated fatty acids include corn, sunflower, sesame and soybean oils. They increase weight because of their high calorie content. A generation ago, polyunsaturates were recommended in preference to saturated fats, which comprised the major fat component of the UK diet. However, although these polyunsaturates are less atherogenic than saturated fat, it is now recommended that they too should be restricted.

Monounsaturated fatty acids are less atherogenic than saturated fats but in excess increase total cholesterol. Common sources include rapeseed, olive and peanut oils, avocados and almonds.

Giving dietary advice

Dietary advice, like all medical advice, should be given with background knowledge of the patient's medical condition; sympathetically; simply, and with enthusiasm and interest. Patients need frequent monitoring and continuing support and encouragement because 'relapse' is common.

It is very important for patients to prove to themselves that they are able to lose weight if they change their eating habits and that they will feel better and fitter and will sleep better after they have lost weight. Patients have to know what it feels like to have lost weight and, if possible, achieve their optimum weight.

Diet clinics in primary care

These are effective and patients generally like them because they have a medical atmosphere and are taken seriously. They are usually run by a nurse and may be organised on a one-to-one level or as a group. They may be part of a cardiovascular prevention clinic.

Methods to maintain weight loss

The most difficult challenge that patients face is maintaining weight loss. Most weight-loss programmes incorporating diet, exercise and behaviour modification result in a 10% weight loss. Most dieters regain about one-third of the weight lost during the next year, and are back to baseline within five years. Continued contact is very important in helping people to maintain weight loss. The most effective way for clinicians to help patients maintain their weight loss is by means of face-to-face consultations. The internet has also been used. Patients should also weigh themselves daily and, if it is not possible for them to be seen in primary care, they may be able to maintain their weight loss by recording their weight and discussing their progress with a clinician by telephone or by email. Weekly contact is helpful.

Aims of a low-fat diet

These include reducing:

❖ total fat intake
❖ saturated fat intake
❖ dietary cholesterol
❖ salt intake
❖ weight.

Reduction of carbohydrate intake in conjunction with reduced fat intake is the initial step in treating type 2 (non-insulin dependent) diabetes.

How to persuade patients to change their eating habits

For many people, the word 'diet' implies deprivation, hardship and suffering. People who tell others that they are on a diet may feel virtuous, brave and proud – all justifiable emotions. Others may feel embarrassed and consider their eating habits private information.

Some patients may find it preferable and less stressful or insulting if dietary recommendations made to lower their cardiovascular risk – for treatment of hypertension or hypercholesterolaemia – are not prescribed as a 'diet' but as suggestions for a long-term modification in their way of eating and living. They may feel this concept is less threatening and depressing. Exercise without dieting does not result in adequate weight loss.

The fundamental failure of diets
- Effective, sustained weight loss is achieved by dietary and nutritional education.
- Long-term weight loss necessitates a permanent modification in a person's eating habits and lifestyle; this is not achieved by short-term 'ceasefires' or diets.
- Diets are, by their nature, temporary reductions in high-calorie eating and drinking.
- As soon as a person stops their diet, their calorie intake increases and their weight gain resumes.
- Diets are the nutritional equivalents of economic 'boom and busts'. That is why there are so many of them and why none of them work in the long term.

Prescribed diets

These are difficult to understand because they recommend limits on dietary components. The National Cholesterol Education Programme (NCEP) diet for primary prevention suggests restrictions of total fat to <30% of energy, saturated fat to <10% of energy, and dietary cholesterol to <200 mg per day. The NCEP diet for patients with vascular disease recommends restricting saturated fat to <7% of energy intake.

The problem with recommendations of this type is that patients may not understand the terms used and what the percentages mean in practice. They need simple advice and this explains the success and popularity of the WeightWatchers™ and Slimmer's World™ diets which are essentially fat and calorie reducing. The weekly weigh-ins with encouragement or criticism are important. Those who do not lose weight or whose weight increases feel guilty and embarrassed. The successful dieters feel proud with their achievement.

Comparison between low-carbohydrate and low-fat diets

The amount of weight loss and its duration depend on the amount and duration of calorie reduction. Patients who are willing to try to lose weight must understand that dieting is a life-long commitment although not necessarily a continual daily burden. The occasional desire to feast is understandable, not life-threatening and, if planned, may be an incentive for the patient both before and after the dietary lapse.

TABLE 7.3 Comparison of low-carbohydrate and low-fat diets

VARIABLE	LOW-CARBOHYDRATE DIET	LOW-FAT DIET
LDL cholesterol	no change	decrease
HDL cholesterol	moderate increase	slight increase
Triglycerides	moderate decrease	slight decrease
Caloric restriction	induced ketosis reduces calorie intake	necessary
Food choices	very restricted	moderately restricted
Rate of weight loss	rapid initially, with diuresis	gradual, with some diuresis
Potential long-term concerns	• calciuria (decreased bone mass and renal stones) • high protein in patients with renal or liver disease • atherogenicity (high fat and low fruit, vegetable and grain intake) • fibre and vitamin deficiency	none

Effect of low-fat diets on lipid levels

Total cholesterol levels fall by approximately 10%, depending on the pre-diet cholesterol intake.

The Mediterranean diet

The benefits of a 'Mediterranean diet' have been recognised since the 1950s. It is based on a diet low in saturated fat but rich in fruit, vegetables, wholegrain cereals, couscous, polenta, bulgar, beans, legumes and nuts, moderate amounts of fish, poultry and wine and occasional red meat. Olive oil is the main source of fat.

The traditional Mediterranean diet is associated with a lower total mortality, coronary mortality and mortality from cancer. The cause for this benefit is unknown but it may be related to a combination of dietary components, olive oil and moderate amounts of wine. People living around the Mediterranean are certainly not uniformly slim or less obese or overweight than people living in Northern Europe. Epidemiological surveys in the early 1950s and 1960s reported a comparatively lower prevalence of coronary heart disease and this was believed to be due to their diet. However, the issue is not clear cut. The prevalence of smoking is now higher among people living in Mediterranean countries because of the smoking bans in many northern European countries, and this may blur or confound any benefits from the Mediterranean diet, which is lower in saturated fats, but which contains considerable amounts of carbohydrates.

The low-fat, high-carbohydrate diet

This is typified in the Asian diet with very low intakes of saturated fat and cholesterol. It results in low total and LDL cholesterol levels.

The low-fat, low-carbohydrate diet

This is a short-term 'no' fat, very low-carbohydrate diet designed for obese patients who may have diabetes, hypertension, hyperlipidaemia and vascular disease. It is simple to understand. Patients can eat as much of the allowed foods as they like. It is a very healthy diet but patients may find it boring. It is particularly useful to help patients 'kick-start' weight loss prior to cardiac surgery or before starting on antihypertensive or diabetic treatment. It is not dangerous and is a slightly more explicit and rigid form of the diet recommended by the British Heart Foundation.

It is restrictive but effective. Patients must be willing and able to stick to a major change in eating habits for at least one month. It should be combined with daily exercise.

Most patients will lose at least 5 kg in the first month, 3 kg in the second and this should continue until the patient achieves their goal weight. Patients should be seen regularly and weighed. When patients have achieved their desired weight, they will need advice about future eating habits. Further supervision reduces the probability of relapse.

The principles of the diet may be continued in the long term and patients can use a strict form of the diet for short periods to reduce their weight when they wish. Patients can stay on the diet for several months although they tend to complain that it is boring, which it is, unless imagination and creativity are used.

Low-fat, low-carbohydrate diets result in significant weight loss and a reduction in total cholesterol, LDL cholesterol and triglycerides.

What is allowed?	There is no restriction on the amount of fish, chicken, salad fruit and vegetables (except potatoes and corn) that can be eaten. The only cheese allowed is very low-fat cottage cheese. Skimmed milk and olive oil may be used for cooking and salads. Patients should drink as much water as they want. Two eggs a week at most is suggested.
What is forbidden?	
Fat:	Butter, cream, saturated fat oils, spreads, mayonnaise, confectionery, chocolate, cheese, sweet desserts.

Carbohydrate: Cereals, sweets, alcohol, crisps, nuts, bread, crackers, biscuits, cakes, potatoes and pasta. Red meat is allowed once per week. Prepared supermarket foods, even the 'low-fat' varieties, may contain high levels of fat and salt which is relevant in patients with hypertension and heart failure.

Low-fat diets rich in fish, fruit, vegetables and whole grains, combined with exercise maintained over a long time have been shown to reduce the rate of death from cardiovascular causes. Fat intake should comprise less than 30% of the total calorie intake.

Patients should be encouraged to cook and prepare their food imaginatively. They are very happy and proud when they lose weight. Constipation is unusual due to the high fibre content and diarrhoea is very unusual. Patients should be monitored and encouraged to continue with the diet until they have achieved their optimal weight or body mass index and, when they do, they can very gradually introduce a small amount of carbohydrate.

After they have achieved their target weight, they may then relax the diet but stick to the main principles and revert to the diet for a few days at a time if their weight drifts up.

The high-protein, high-fat, low-carbohydrate diet

This is currently fashionable and is the principle of the previously popular 'Dr Atkins' diet'. Like most diets, it is effective in some patients who like the freedom and encouragement to eat protein and fat while reducing total calorie intake. The diet allows unlimited fat and protein but prohibits carbohydrate and fruit and vegetables. Not surprisingly, it increases the cholesterol and triglyceride levels and this is very undesirable in patients with coronary artery disease or who are at risk of developing coronary artery disease. Patients often complain of unpleasant constipation and wind. Weight loss with these diets is due to the duration of the diet and the restriction of calories but not due to the reduction in carbohydrate intake alone.

Two recent studies have shown that compared with a traditional low-fat diet (less than 30% of the total calorie intake), a low-carbohydrate diet followed for 90 days resulted in a greater weight loss. After one year, there was no significant difference in the weight between the groups of patients in the two groups, probably because of non-compliance and this highlights the well-known difficulty that people, particularly those who are obese and who have a fondness for food, have in maintaining a healthy eating habit. The potential problems of a long-term low-carbohydrate, high-fat and high-protein diet are shown above in Table 7.3. Nevertheless, the dangers of severe obesity probably outweigh those of the diet in a slim and otherwise healthy person.

It is important to ask all patients if they are on a particular diet or whether they take any dietary supplements – conventional or homoeopathic. Supplements may have 'an effect' in lowering cholesterol but this may not translate into a reduction in coronary heart disease.

Fish oils

Oils found in oily fish (salmon, mackerel, swordfish) contain n-3 fatty acids which may provide protection against cardiovascular disease possibly by reducing ventricular arrhythmias and sudden death. There may be other benefits of oily fish on triglycerides, blood pressure and clotting mechanisms. It is recommended that oily fish be eaten at least twice a week.

Dietary fibre

This is an important part of a balanced diet. Insoluble fibre is roughage and reduces constipation. Sources high in insoluble fibre are blackberries, beans, parsnips, pears, wholegrain bread and wheat bran. Soluble fibre is contained in oatbran, dried beans, grains, green vegetables and fruit. It reduces total and LDL cholesterol by altering bile acid metabolism.

Soya protein

This lowers cholesterol but the mechanism is unclear. It contains isoflavanoids and antioxidants and may affect platelets and thrombin.

Coffee

Boiled coffee increases total and LDL cholesterol levels due to the alcohols in the oil droplets called cafestol and kahweol. Although drinking more than five cups of coffee per day has been shown to increase the risk of coronary artery disease, drinking one or two cups per day probably has no effect on either lipid levels or coronary heart disease rates.

Garlic

One half to one whole clove of garlic per day decreases total cholesterol by 9% but there is no good evidence that garlic has any beneficial effect on coronary heart disease.

Alcohol and the red wine hypothesis

Alcohol is calorific, fattening, increases triglycerides and HDL, and also increases blood pressure. In excess it leads to hypertension, cardiomyopathy and arrhythmia (ectopics and atrial fibrillation). In excess it has several other damaging effects on the body.

Moderate alcohol consumption – one to two units per day – decreases cardiovascular mortality. It was suggested that red wine might explain the low cardiac mortality in France (the so-called 'French paradox'). The French eat quite a lot of fat including cheese but the population has high HDL levels. Red wine contains polyphenols including resveratrol, which when isolated from alcohol and given to animals has protective effects against ischaemia. These include decreased arterial damage to ischaemia, decreased activity of angiotensin II, increases in nitric oxide (a vasodilator), increased endogenous tissue plasminogen activator and lower fibrinogen levels with decreased platelet aggregation reducing the tendency to thrombosis. Alcohol in moderation increases protective HDL levels. There is no evidence that red wine is superior to white wine as a cardioprotective agent.

Alcohol in moderation appears to exert a more striking beneficial effect in women.

Drug treatment

Drug treatment for obesity is considered by the National Institute for Clinical Effectiveness to be cost effective. Drug treatment for obesity should be started if patients remain dangerously obese, with a BMI of 30 kg/m^2 despite a supervised three-month diet and exercise programme. Patients who have adhered to this preferred, first-line treatment should lose weight. It may be appropriate to prescribe anti-obesity drugs to patients with a BMI of <27 kg/m^2 if they have associated cardiovascular risk factors. Anti-obesity drugs should be stopped if patients do not lose more than 5% of their baseline weight. Patients should be monitored carefully while on medication to see if they have side effects.

Most drugs are licensed to be used for three months and continued only if the person has lost at least 5% of their initial body weight since starting treatment. Diet drugs generally should not be prescribed for longer than two years. They may be used to help maintain weight loss.

Obesity is often associated with depression and psychological disturbances and all these aspects need careful assessment and treatment.

Anti-obesity drugs:
- ◇ induce a further 5 kg weight loss compared with diet alone
- ◇ maintain weight loss 12 kg below baseline
- ◇ improve cardiovascular risk factors due to weight loss
- ◇ should not be used in combination with other anti-obesity drugs
- ◇ should be used in combination with diet and exercise
- ◇ should be stopped if the individual puts on weight during treatment.

Drugs not recommended for treating obesity

Dexfenfluramine, fenfluramine and amphetamines should no longer be prescribed for obesity. They cause pulmonary hypertension and valvular heart disease. There is no evidence that methylcellulose is effective or safe. Phentermine is a catecholamine-releasing agent stimulating the central nervous system causing appetite suppression. It should not be prescribed because its efficacy and safety have not been established.

Thyroid hormones should not be used to treat obesity, except in patients with biochemical hypothyroidism. Diuretics and amphetamine should not be used to treat obesity.

Sibutramine

This drug has been licensed for the treatment of obese patients with a body mass index of >30 kg/m^2 and for patients with a body mass index of 27 kg/m^2 if they have diabetes or dyslipidaemias. It inhibits the re-uptake of noradrenaline and serotonin in the brain and so reduces appetite. It is the preferred drug for patients who cannot control their eating habits. It is contraindicated in patients with a history of a major eating disorder, or psychiatric disorder, or heart failure.

Most patients take 10 mg once a day. The dose can be increased if weight loss is less than 2 kg after four weeks. It should be used as part of a weight-reducing programme combined with exercise and a low-calorie diet.

It can be expected to result in a 5–10% weight loss in the majority of patients. There are associated benefits in lipid profile with the HDL-cholesterol increasing by 25%. The noradrenergic effects tend to increase blood pressure and so the blood pressure must be monitored. Patients should be offered support and advice during treatment. It should be stopped if the blood pressure increases above 140/95 mmHg. Controlled hypertension is not a contraindication to prescribing sibutramine.

There are many side effects including dry mouth, constipation, headaches, dizziness, poor sleep, agitation and arrhythmia.

It should be used with caution in patients with arrhythmias and coronary heart disease and is contraindicated in patients with recent myocardial infarction (less than six weeks). Blood pressure and pulse rate should be recorded two-weekly during the first three months, monthly for the next three months and then every three months.

Sibutramine should be stopped if there is no response defined as less than 5% weight loss from baseline after three months, or if individuals put on weight, or if the blood pressure increases above 145/90 mmHg or by more than 10%.

Orlistat

Orlistat is a lipase inhibitor, reducing the absorption of around 30% of dietary fat. Non-absorption of 20 g of fat per day is the equivalent of a reduction of 180 Kcal per day.

It should be used for no more than three months unless there has been at least a 5% weight loss. It may impair absorption of fat-soluble vitamins and so multivitamins may be needed and should be taken two hours after the orlistat dose or at bedtime. It is contraindicated in chronic malabsorption syndrome.

Side effects include wind, oily leak from the rectum, liquid stools, faecal incontinence, abdominal distension and pain, fatigue, headache.

The dose is 120 mg taken immediately before, during or up to one hour after each meal to a maximum daily dose of 360 mg. The dose should be omitted if the meal contains little or no fat. Patients who continue to eat a lot of fat will have steatorrhea. Orlistat should not be used with other types of diet drug.

Rimonabant (Acomplia)

Cannabis inhalation induces hunger ('the munchies'). Blocking cannabinoid receptors in the brain suppresses appetite. Rimonabant is the first cannabinoid-1 receptor antagonist licensed for treating obesity. It is indicated as an adjunct to diet and exercise for the treatment of obese patients (BMI ≥30 kg/m^2), or overweight patients (>27 kg/m^2) with associated risk factor(s), such as type 2 diabetes or dyslipidaemia.

Its use results in weight loss and improvement in some cardiovascular risk factors. There is a 5–10% weight loss in most patients, which is maintained for two years.

Side effects are mild and include nausea and depression.

Rimonabant is contraindicated in patients with depression and suicidal behaviour and should not be prescribed to patients with ongoing major depressive illness and/or ongoing treatment with antidepressants, unless the benefit of the treatment is considered to outweigh the potential risks.

In clinical trials, depressive disorders or mood alterations with depressive symptoms have been reported in up to 10%, and suicidal ideation in up to 1%, of patients receiving rimonabant. This risk may be increased in patients with a past history of psychiatric illness. Patients and carers or relatives should be informed about the risk of depression. Patients should be encouraged to stop treatment and seek medical advice if symptoms of depression occur. Rimonabant should be stopped if depression occurs.

Surgical treatment for obesity: 'bariatric' surgery

This is performed only rarely in the UK, for several reasons. GPs and hospital doctors know little about its effects and patients consider it drastic and dangerous and may not want their friends and family to know that they were unable to lose weight by changing their eating habits. There are few centres in the UK NHS offering this form of treatment.

Because of the increasing prevalence of obesity, it is possible that more patients will be referred for bariatric surgery if the long term results show that it is safe and cost-effective long-term.

Bariatric surgery for severe obesity, combined with changes in eating habits and long-term monitoring and support, has a role in the management of patients with severe obesity, where the risks of obesity and its complications outweigh the risks of surgery. Bariatric surgery has been shown to be superior to dieting in reducing weight, all-cause mortality, mortality due to cancer and cardiovascular mortality. These benefits in weight reduction are sustained in the long term.

All the following criteria should be fulfilled if bariatric surgery is to be offered to a patient.

✧ The BMI should be >40 kg/m² or >35 kg/m² if they are diabetic or hypertensive.
✧ All non-surgical avenues must have been explored but have failed.
✧ The person will be followed up in a unit with staff experienced in this specialty.
✧ The person is physically and psychologically fit for a general anaesthetic and surgery.
✧ The person commits to long-term follow-up.

Patients have to be carefully assessed and the procedures explained to them in detail, by experienced staff working in a centre with good surgical results. There are significant risks of surgery. For surgical procedures, and not including endoscopic gastric banding, mortality at one year ranges from 11% in patients aged over 65 years to 4% in younger people. Morbidity and mortality increase in older patients with more associated medical complications, or who have more disruptive procedures. Patients should have a comprehensive risk evaluation before surgery. The most appropriate intervention should be chosen by the specialist and the patient.

Overall morbidity is 14% due to myocardial infarction, infection, bleeding, thromboembolism, wound complications, chest infections. Two per cent of patients require a second operation. Digestive problems remain a problem in 36% of patients five years post-operatively.

Bariatric surgery is not generally recommended for children.

Operative aims

There are two main approaches:
1. to reduce energy intake and absorption and increase energy output
2. to make patients feel fuller and reduce their appetite and so reduce their calorie intake.

Bariatric surgical procedures

There are several types of operation:
*   gastric banding, which is done endoscopically
*   gastric bypass
*   vertical banded gastroplasty
*   biliary-pancreatic diversion
*   sleeve gastrectomy.

Advice for patients

*   Obesity is dangerous and increases the risk of heart attack, stroke and several other medical conditions.
*   Obese people do not live as long as slim people.
*   When you are slim and fit, you will feel better, look better and live longer.
*   Good eating and exercise habits, together with the habit of not smoking, start in childhood.
*   A healthy diet and maintenance of an optimum weight is important. Eating a healthy diet, not smoking and doing regular exercise, reduce your risk of heart disease, diabetes and several other conditions including cancer. These sensible daily habits increase your chances of living a longer life.
*   The less food and calories you eat and drink, the more weight you will lose.
*   The quickest way to lose weight is a no-fat, very low-carbohydrate diet having plenty of natural food – salad, fruit and fresh vegetables, fish and moderate amounts of meat. It is difficult but effective.
*   Alcohol is fattening. The risks outweigh any small benefits. There is some evidence that a small amount of red wine is beneficial in some people. If you are overweight, you should not drink any alcohol, or at most, perhaps, one unit per day.
*   Ready-to-cook meals contain large amounts of salt and fat.
*   All fast food, sandwiches, pizza, hamburgers, fried chicken, and take-away foods are high in calories. If you are overweight, you should eat only fresh, nutritious food.

Salad, fruit and non-starchy vegetables contain very few calories. You can eat as much of these as you want.

✧ Restaurants use large amounts of salt and fat, particularly butter.

✧ A key part of a healthy diet is reducing the amount of fat you eat. Try to avoid saturated fat (butter, cream, cheese; all other dairy food; fast food; animal fat – for example, red fatty meat – more than once a week; food cooked in fat – crisps, chips, deep-fried food; chocolate; eggs, liver).

✧ Starch – bread (any bread, including wholemeal and organic bread), potatoes, rice, pasta, food containing flour, corn – is fattening.

✧ Avoid salt and salty food.

✧ Once you have started to lose weight, weigh yourself daily and plan your day and the meals you eat. Avoid snacking unless you eat fruit and vegetables. Do not eat fast foods because you are rushed and hungry. Eat good food, before you get hungry.

Answers to questions about clinical cases

1. She should not go on to the Atkins diet. This is a very high-fat diet which increases the blood cholesterol. She should instead be advised to have a conventional low-fat, high-fibre diet eating fruit, vegetables and fish and chicken. A small amount of alcohol is acceptable but this will reduce the speed of her weight loss.

2. If you are not sure about the diagnosis, contact the consultant or the registrar, to make sure that the patient had unstable angina, and not oesophageal pain. Tell him that moderate wine consumption is acceptable and might be good for him but that drinking one bottle per day is too much. One glass is quite enough. He should have a cardiovascular risk assessment, including a dietary history, weight, blood pressure, blood tests for fasting lipids, glucose, full blood count, renal function, liver function, and exercise testing. Check his cardiac medications. If he can tolerate these medications he should be on aspirin, a β-blocker, a statin, possibly an ACE inhibitor. He should be advised about diet, weight, stress management, and exercise. He may already have had or be scheduled for coronary angiography and this will provide the information he wants about the reasons for his recent heart problem.

3. He appears keen to reduce his cardiovascular risk. Anyone who succeeds in stopping smoking should be able, with help and support, to change their eating habits. Discuss various dietary approaches, point out specifically the potential benefits and either enrol him into a cardiovascular prevention clinic at your surgery or, if possible, see him yourself until he is on the right path. He will need continual supervision. All other cardiovascular prevention measures, including exercise, are important.

4. This is a common and difficult problem. A medical cause of obesity should be excluded and it may be necessary for the whole family to be seen. If the cause of obesity is due solely to an inappropriate high-calorie diet, the family should be asked if they want to lose weight. If they do not want to change their eating habits, then there is little a doctor can do to impose sound medical advice on the family. If the family members are genuinely keen to lose weight and would welcome advice and dietary education, then a full programme should be offered. This is difficult, time consuming

and requires enthusiastic staff who are able and willing to provide a long-term service. It will require a carefully thought-out, simple, direct and accessible clinical and psychological support service for this major public health problem. It should be part of a comprehensive cardiovascular prevention service offered to patients of all ages.

5. She has proved to herself and you that she is able to lose weight and has the willpower and ability to do so. The key issue is whether she understands why she puts on weight (in her case a love of ice-cream and large portions of food), and whether she would be emotionally stable enough for long enough to lose weight on a simple low-calorie diet, combined with sensible tailored exercise. This has to be discussed and she needs to tell you what she would like to do and how she would like to do it. She will not lose weight unless she really wants to do so. Regular consultations, weighing, interest, compassion, reminding her of her hypertension and the other risks of obesity, will help. She needs to establish an eating habit that she can live with in the long term.

6. She has been successful on WeightWatchers™ in the past. This, together with daily exercise, is what she should try first. If she is unsuccessful, and if her BMI exceeds 30 kg/m^2, or 27 kg/m^2 and she has cardiovascular risk factors, then she should have a trial of an anti-obesity drug. It doesn't matter which one is tried first, but she must understand that she will remain overweight, despite the tablet, unless she makes permanent changes to her dietary habits to maintain her weight loss. She will need monitoring and frequent face-to-face consultations with a member of the primary care team she respects. If all else fails and she remains dangerously obese, bariatric surgery should be considered and she should be referred to an experienced centre for evaluation.

FURTHER READING

Albert CM, Campos H, Stampfer MJ, *et al.* Blood levels of long-chain n-3 fatty acids and the risk of sudden death. *N Engl J Med.* 2002; **346:** 1113–18.

Alberti K, Zimmet P. Definition, diagnosis and classification of diabetes mellitus and its complications. Part I: diagnosis and classification of diabetes mellitus provisional report of a WHO consultation. *Diabetic Med.* 1998; **15:** 539–53.

American College of Obstetricians and Gynecologists. *Guidance on the impact of obesity on pregnancy.* 2005. Available at: www.acog.org/from_home/publications/press_releases/nr08-31-05-2.cfm.

Barsch GS, Farooqi IS, O'Rahilly S. Genetics of body-weight regulation. *Nature.* 2000; **404:** 644–51.

BMJ Clinical Evidence. Available at: www.clinicalevidence.com/ceweb/conditions/end/0604/0604_17.jsp (accessed February 2007).

Bravata DM, Sanders L, Huang J, *et al.* Efficacy and safety of low-carbohydrate diets: a systematic review. *JAMA.* 2003; **289:** 1837–50.

Colquitt J, Clegg A, Loveman E, *et al. Surgery of morbid obesity* (Cochrane Review). The Cochrane Library, Issue 4. Chichester, UK: John Wiley & Sons; 2005.

de Koning L, Merchant AT, Pogue J, Anand SS. Waist circumference and waist-to-hip ratio as predictors of cardiovascular events: meta-regression analysis of prospective studies. *Eur Heart J.* 2007; **28:** 850–6.

Finer N (2005). Does pharmacologically-induced weight loss improve cardiovascular outcome? Impact of anti-obesity agents on cardiovascular risk. *Eur Heart J.* 2005; **7(Suppl.):** L32–8.

Foster GD, Wyatt HR, Hill JO, *et al.* A randomised trial of a low-carbohydrate diet for obesity. *N Engl J Med.* 2003; **348:** 2082–90.

Garson A Jr, Engelhard CL (2007). Attacking obesity: lessons from smoking. *J Am Coll Cardiol.* 2007; **49:** 1673–5.

Handler C, Coghlan G. *Living with Coronary Disease.* London: Springer; 2007.

Institute of Medicine (US). *Progress in preventing childhood obesity: how do we measure up?* Washington, DC: National Academies of Sciences; 2006.

International Diabetes Federation. *The IDF consensus worldwide definition of the metabolic syndrome.* 2005. Available at: www.idf.org/webdata/docs/Metacsyndrome/def.pdf

James WPT, Astrup A, Finer N, *et al.* for the STORM Study Group. Effect of sibutramine on weight maintenance after weight loss: a randomised trial. *Lancet.* 2000; **356:** 2119–25.

Kenchaiah S, Evans JC, Levy D, *et al.* Obesity and the risk of heart failure. *N Engl J Med.* 2002; **347:** 305–13.

Keys A, *et al. Seven Countries: A multivariate analysis of death and coronary heart disease.* Cambridge, MA: Harvard University Press; 1980. pp. 1–381.

LaCroix AZ, Mead LA, Liang KY, *et al.* Coffee consumption and the incidence of coronary heart disease. *N Engl J Med.* 1986; **315:** 377–82.

Maggard MA, Shugarman LR, Suttorp M, *et al.* Meta-analysis: surgical treatment of obesity. *Ann Intern Med.* 2005; **142:** 547–59.

Mello MM, Studdert DM, Brennan TA. Obesity – the new frontier of public health law. *N Engl J Med.* 2006; **354:** 2601–10.

Must A, Spadano J, Coakley EH, *et al.* The disease burden associated with overweight and obesity. *JAMA.* 1999; **282:** 1523–9.

National Cholesterol Education Program. Executive Summary of the Third Report of the National Cholesterol Education Program (NCEP) Expert Panel on Detection, Evaluation, and Treatment of High Blood Cholesterol in Adults (Adult Treatment Panel III). *JAMA.* 2001; **285:** 2486–97.

National Cholesterol Education Program. *Report of the expert panel on population strategies for blood cholesterol reduction.* US Dept of Health and Human Services; 1990. Publication NIH 90-3046.

National Heart, Lung and Blood Institute. *The practical guide: identification, evaluation, and treatment of overweight and obesity in adult.* 2006. Available at: www.nhlbi.nih.gov/guideline/obesity/practgde.htm.

Royal College of Physicians. *Report: Clinical management of overweight and obese patients with particular reference to the use of drugs.* The Royal College of Physicians, London; 1998.

Samaha FF, Iqbal N, Sesadri P, *et al.* A low-carbohydrate as compared with a low-fat diet in severe obesity. *N Engl J Med.* 2003; **348:** 2074–81.

Sjostrom L, Lindroos AK, Peltonen M, *et al.*, and The Swedish Obese Subjects Study Group. Lifestyle, diabetes, and cardiovascular risk factors 10 years after bariatric surgery. *N Engl J Med.* 2004; **351:** 2683–93.

Trichopoulou A, Costacou T, Bamia C, Trichopoulos D. Adherence to a Mediterranean diet and survival in Greek population. *N Engl J Med.* 2003; **348:** 2599–608.

Wing RR, Tate DF, Gorin AA, Raynor HA, Fava JL. A self-regulation program for maintenance of weight loss. *N Engl J Med.* 2006; **355:** 1563–71.

Wirth A, Krause J. Long-term weight loss with Sibutramine: a randomised controlled trial. *JAMA.* 2001; **286:** 1331–9.

World Health Organization. *Global strategy on diet, physical activity and health.* 2006. Available at: www.who.int/dietphysicalactivity/publications/facts/obesity/.

Smoking

EIGHT

Clinical cases

1. An 81-year-old man who has smoked 40 cigarettes a day for at least 60 years and who is hypertensive with a previous transient ischaemic attack comes to your surgery complaining of chest pain. Apart from reviewing his treatment for hypertension, checking his blood pressure, checking his diabetic status and advising him to stop smoking, what else do you do?
2. A 43-year-old man attends your surgery two weeks after a heart attack. He is symptom free and has not been able to stop smoking and would like help from you. What do you do?
3. A 64-year-old female with cor pulmonale and chronic obstructive airways disease comes to see you with a chest infection. What do you do?
4. An 18-year-old girl who smokes 10 cigarettes per day wants to start the oral contraceptive pill. What do you do?
5. A 52-year-old woman with a long history of depression, alcoholism and previous oesophageal pain and who smokes 30 cigarettes per day, comes to see you complaining of chest pain. What do you do?

Nicotine

Nicotine, the addictive alkaloid component of tobacco, is thought to have been named after Jean Nicot, a sixteenth-century French Ambassador to Portugal, who believed and promoted the idea that tobacco had curative powers although it is not clear why he thought this. Certainly, ideas like this would be more rigorously tested today.

Prevalence and risks

An estimated 13 million people smoke in Britain, with an equal proportion of male and females (25% of each). Smoking is more prevalent in people of lower socio-economic class and lower educational status. It is becoming more common in young girls and boys and so school education and prevention programmes are important. Smoking can become an addiction shortly after a person starts the habit.

Smoking is the single largest cause of death, disability, preventable illness and unnecessary health expense in the UK. It is a direct cause of cancer of the lung, larynx, mouth, oesophagus and bladder. It contributes to the development of cancer of the kidney, bladder, pancreas and cervix. It is the main cause of chronic obstructive pulmonary disease which may result in right heart failure. It has been estimated to cause between 17% and 30% of all cardiovascular deaths. Smoking shortens the lifespan by an estimated 10 years. About 50% of smokers die from a smoking-related illness.

In smokers, the cardiovascular risk increases by 25%. Lung cancer risk increases by 30%.

Smoking and cardiovascular disease

Cardiovascular disease is the most common smoking-related cause of death. In the 35- to 69-year age group, 25% of deaths are due to tobacco. Middle-aged men who smoke more than 20 cigarettes per day are at two to three times greater risk of having a major cardiac event or sudden death than are non-smokers.

The risk for developing coronary heart disease is dose related. The damage to the cardiovascular system increases with the number of cigarettes smoked, and the dose of nicotine absorbed, which is related to the depth of inhalation.

Even one cigarette per day, particularly in women, doubles the risk of cardiovascular disease. The cardiovascular morbidity and mortality risks for women are similar to those for men, but the risk of fatal myocardial infarction is 13 times greater if they use the oral contraceptive pill.

Second-hand smoke increases the risk of cardiovascular disease by 30%, and is an important cause of non-cardiac diseases. Tobacco acts synergistically with other cardiovascular risk factors.

Benefits of smoking cessation

A person who stops smoking halves their risk of coronary heart disease and coronary events, including death, within one year. This benefit occurs in people of all ages. After 15 years of smoking cessation, their cardiovascular and other risks are similar to those of a person who has never smoked. However, there is a substantial risk reduction four years after smoking cessation. This benefit applies to smokers of all ages.

Smoking cessation in patients with coronary heart disease reduces cardiovascular risk by 36%, similar to the risk reduction resulting from statins in high-risk individuals. Smoking cessation combined with statins exerts a powerful secondary preventive effect.

Smoking cessation reduces restenosis after coronary angioplasty, and reduces graft stenosis after coronary artery surgery and peripheral vascular surgery.

In patients with heart failure, smoking cessation reduces mortality by as much as, or more than, treatment with β-blockers, aldosterone antagonists, or angiotensin-converting enzyme inhibitors.

Erectile dysfunction may improve within one month of smoking cessation.

The risks of cancer and chronic obstructive pulmonary disease both fall to near non-smoker levels progressively after smoking cessation.

Smoking cessation should be the main focus of risk reduction for patients with vascular disease. The management of nicotine addiction is similar to the management of heroin and cocaine addiction. Stopping smoking reduces the 10-year risk of death by more than half (54% to 18%). It is the single most important cardiovascular intervention conferring the greatest symptomatic and prognostic benefit. Patients who continue to smoke have a three times greater risk of death compared with those who quit.

Smoking cessation and statins have similar benefits in reducing cardiovascular risk in patients with coronary heart disease.

Smoking cessation, if achieved without the use of medication or prolonged counselling, is the most cost-effective cardiovascular disease prevention measure.

Smoking and attributable risk in young adults

Smoking is more dangerous in young people than it is in older people. Smoking is the main cause of heart attacks in patients aged less than 50 years.

Benefits of never smoking

Men and women who never smoke live 6.2 and 4.9 years longer, respectively, compared with smokers. This is because of their reduced risk of cardiovascular and other conditions.

Effects of nicotine on atherogenesis and the cardiovascular system

The effects of cigarette smoke on arterial endothelium and bronchial smooth muscle occur within a few minutes of exposure. The benefits of stopping smoking also occur quite quickly.

1. Effects of nicotine on atherosclerosis

- Direct damage to arterial endothelium.
- Reduced nitric oxide production.
- Depletion of antioxidants.
- Increased smooth muscle proliferation.
- Endothelial inflammation.
- Plaque formation, plaque rupture.
- Reduced endothelial-dependent vasodilatation.
- Reduced HDL cholesterol levels.
- Increased LDL cholesterol levels.

2. Effects of nicotine on thrombosis

- Increased platelet stickiness.
- Increased fibrinogen.
- Increased plasma viscosity.
- Increased arterial wall stiffness and tendency for plaque rupture.

3. Effects of nicotine on coronary artery spasm

- Coronary vasoconstriction.

4. Effects of nicotine on arrhythmias
✧ Increased cathecholamine levels
✧ Decreased threshold for arrhythmias.
✧ Increased oxygen demand.
✧ Reduces oxygen-carrying capacity.

5. Effects of nicotine on arteries
✧ Peripheral vascular disease.
✧ Coronary heart disease.
✧ Carotid artery disease.
✧ Cerebrovascular disease.
✧ Aortic aneurysm.
✧ Renal artery stenosis.
✧ Erectile dysfunction.

6. Haemodynamic effects of nicotine
✧ Acute increase in blood pressure.
✧ Acute increase in heart rate.
✧ Increase in myocardial oxygen demand.
✧ Reduced oxygen carrying capacity of blood with increase in carboxyhaemoglobin.

Cigars, pipes and filter cigarettes
Cigars
Cigar smokers are at similar risk as cigarette smokers. It is difficult to estimate the risk of cigar smoking because cigars vary in length and tobacco content and some cigar smokers inhale while others do not.

Pipe smokers and tobacco chewers
There is no evidence that pipe smokers are at lower risk from cardiovascular disease compared with cigarette smokers. Pipe smokers may be at greater risk because of the amount of nicotine smoked in each pipe and the length of time the person keeps sucking and inhaling on the pipe. Pipe smokers and tobacco chewers are at high risk from cancer of the mouth and tongue.

Smoking filters and low-tar cigarettes
There is no evidence that cigarettes with filters or low-tar cigarettes are less harmful than non-filter-tipped cigarettes. The quantities of carbon monoxide and other noxious chemicals and gases are similar.

Difficulties of smoking cessation
Addiction and withdrawal symptoms
Nicotine is highly addictive. In approximately 50% of people, tobacco withdrawal results in depression, insomnia, irritability, anxiety, difficulty in concentration, restlessness, and increased appetite and weight gain. The symptoms appear within a few hours, peak at one to two days and last for at least several weeks – and in some people, for many months. This explains why only 5% of smokers are still non-smokers one year after they attempt to quit.

Weight gain
Most people gain at least 3 kg and some much more. Fear of weight gain is a potent deterrent for people, particularly women, to stop smoking and so this needs to be addressed in smoking cessation programmes which should, where appropriate, address all risk factors.

Role of primary care physicians in smoking cessation
A smoking cessation programme is an important primary care service with great primary and secondary cardiac prevention and general health benefits. Ideally it should be combined with other cardiac risk-factor interventions. Practices may wish to set up a telephone help and support line.

Partners, spouses, relatives, work colleagues and schoolfriends
The influence of other smokers on the smoking habits of the patient is difficult to quantify but should not be underestimated. There is little data on this. Understandably, smokers find it exceptionally difficult to stop smoking even with motivation if they are in close contact at home or at work with other smokers who may feel resentful if told that they, too, should stop smoking. Peer pressure among schoolchildren is a well-recognised and powerful influence inducing children to smoke.

Smoking cessation programmes
Motivational support programmes increase the chances of successful quitting. Unfortunately, however, smoking cessation programmes and treatments have a very low success rate and success ultimately depends on the smoker wanting to stop smoking and making a serious, sustained effort and being prepared to suffer the withdrawal symptoms which can last for a long time. Some quitters claim that the desire to smoke is always there.

It is insufficient to simply advise patients to stop smoking. A two-minute 'lecture' or admonishment by a doctor has little long-term effect. The success of a consultation advising patients to stop smoking depends on how the message is conveyed to the patient and, most importantly, on the patient's willingness and their motivation to stop. Patients are more likely to stop smoking after a heart attack or coronary angiography showing important coronary artery disease necessitating myocardial revascularisation.

Smoking cessation advice given by more than one primary care health provider is more effective than if only one clinician is involved. Success rates improve when additional advice is provided by a specialist and when intense, frequent and prolonged sessions are provided. The resource implications are substantial and need to be supported.

The recent smoking ban in public places prohibits people smoking in restaurants, wine bars, pubs, other public places and in the workplace. Although the effect the ban will have on the prevalence of smoking is not yet known, it seems likely that the number of smokers will reduce.

The '4As' primary care approach to help patients stop smoking

ASK   identify smokers in the practice.

ADVISE   strongly advise all smokers to stop and explain the risks of continuance and the benefits of stopping.

ASSIST   set a stop date, offer nicotine replacement, offer smoking cessation clinic, offer written supplemental materials, offer motivational advice, encourage relatives and friends to offer support and encouragement.

ARRANGE   follow-up advice and clinics.

Patients know that smoking is dangerous, but – even after a heart attack – find it difficult to stop smoking completely and forever. Patients who fail to quit are often embarrassed about what they think might be perceived as a character failing, and so may not admit that they continue to smoke. It is important to try to identify these patients and offer them help.

Success of smoking cessation clinics

Patients should be helped with a smoking cessation programme combining group, drug and behavioural therapy. This combined approach results in 40% of participants stopping smoking for at least one year. This programme can be led by suitably trained, enthusiastic staff who may have quit smoking successfully. A joint collaborative programme could be established between neighbouring practices.

Help the patients overcome their perceived obstacles to stopping smoking. These include stress at home and/or at work, personal problems, the fear of weight gain, and the fear of withdrawal symptoms. The benefits of stopping and the risks and costs of not stopping should be reiterated but in a positive and sympathetic manner.

> Nicotine replacement and bupropion, combined with some form of behavioural support, are recommended as first-line treatments but only for patients who commit to a target stop date. These treatments should be combined with advice and encouragement to stop.

Nicotine replacement

Nicotine replacement treatment improves the smoking cessation rate. Patient preferences for gum, skin patches and nasal spray, inhaler, lozenges and sublingual tablets, differ. Most forms of nicotine replacement therapies are available over the counter. They should be used at regular intervals and also to relieve sudden cravings for nicotine. They are safe and can be taken by patients with cardiovascular disease. Prescribe the form of nicotine replacement the patient finds most acceptable. There are no important contraindications to its use.

Nicotine gum should be chewed slowly until a peppery or mint taste emerges and then parked between the cheek and the mucosa. It should be alternatively chewed and parked for 30 minutes until the taste disappears. Patients can chew up to 24 pieces of gum per day. Acid drinks, coffee, wine and fruit juices lower the pH in the mouth, theoretically reducing nicotine absorption. The gum can stick to bridges, fillings, dentures and crowns. Nicotine lozenges provide a higher nicotine dose than gum.

The long-term success of nicotine patches in helping smokers stop smoking is low. Nicotine doubles the chances of a smoker remaining smoke free, whether used alone or as part of a formal quit programme. Only 5% of people remain abstinent from smoking eight years after using a nicotine patch for a single 12-week treatment period.

There is some interest in the theoretical advantages of a 'nicotine vaccine' but there is no clinical information on this.

Bupropion (amfebutamone)

Bupropion is an antidepressant with noradrenergic and dopaminergic activity. It is a non-nicotine-based treatment for use in smoking cessation. It increases noradrenaline and dopamine levels in the brain. Its mode of action as an aid for smoking cessation is not clear.

It is effective for those who smoke more than 10 cigarettes per day and is well tolerated. It is equally effective as nicotine replacement and significantly more effective than placebo as an aid to stopping smoking at one year of follow-up after an eight-week treatment period. It has been recommended as an aid to smoking cessation by the National Institute for Clinical Excellence and is available on an NHS prescription. It does not appear to affect blood pressure despite its mode of action.

It is recommended for smokers who are particularly refractory to other treatment. The recommended dose is 150 mg twice a day, usually for seven weeks. Bupropion 150 mg once a day is recommended for elderly patients and those who may be prone to seizures. The incidence of seizures is 0.1%. Other adverse effects include angioedema. It should be started a week or two before intended smoking cessation and continued for two to three months.

There are contraindications to its use in around one-third of potential patients. These include epileptics, those with an eating disorder, and those with a tendency to seizures. It has no significant cardiovascular side effects and can be used in patients with coronary artery disease. It is contraindicated in patients on drugs which lower seizure threshold. These include antidepressants, antimalarials, antipsychotics, corticosteroids, excess alcohol consumption, sedatives and antihistamines.

When used in conjunction with group and individual counselling techniques, bupropion is twice as effective as a placebo in helping patients to quit smoking. Side effects include a dry mouth and insomnia and it is contraindicated in patients with epilepsy, psychosis or who suffer from severe panic disorders.

The indications for bupropion include:

✧ motivated addicted smokers keen to quit
✧ nicotine dependence
✧ patients involved in a support programme.

Nortryptiline

This tricyclic antidepressant is a second-line drug, because of associated side effects. These include dry mouth, difficulty in focusing, glaucoma, constipation, problems for men in passing urine, arrhythmias, postural hypotension, sweating, tremor, and interference with sexual function.

Newer treatments

Rimonabant

The endocannabinoid system is over-activated in smokers. Rimonabant is a cannabinoid receptor blocker. It is licensed for treating obesity, a common consequence of smoking cessation and for many smokers, a reason for their reluctance to quit. There is little information on its use in smoking cessation.

Varenicline

This is a nicotine receptor agonist. It is available in Europe, the USA and on prescription in the UK. Small studies suggest that it is at least as effective as buproprion. It reduces the urge to smoke and nicotine craving by reducing the nicotine 'reward pathways' in the brain which are thought to play a part in nicotine addiction. It has no contraindications.

Side effects include nausea, insomnia, dreams and altered taste.

Clonidine

Clonidine is an α-blocker used in treating hypertension. It has been used to dampen nicotine withdrawal in doses of 0.1 mg to 0.4 mg per day for two to six weeks. It is indicated for people who prefer not to receive nicotine replacement. It can be used in both oral and patch forms. The side effects include sedation, dry mouth and postural hypotension.

Unproven complementary treatments

The Cochrane group found that hypnotherapy, acupuncture and aversion therapy to have no significant effect.

The future

Although prevention is better than cure, it is unlikely that the sale of tobacco will be made illegal. The smoking ban introduced in England in 2007 is likely to encourage smokers to quit but this is not yet established. Because tobacco advertising increases tobacco consumption in young people, a ban on all tobacco advertising and a programme of education in schools and colleges would probably be effective.

Advice for patients

- The nicotine, tar and carbon monoxide in cigarettes are very dangerous and cause irreparable damage to your heart, all your arteries and your lungs.
- Stopping smoking is more important than anything else you can do yourself to improve your health and reduce your risks of having a heart attack, a stroke or lung cancer. Your health will improve from the day you stop.
- We understand how difficult it is and we will help you.
- Even though we are willing to help you, it is something that you have to want to do and do for yourself and your family.
- If you smoke after a heart bypass, or balloon angioplasty or heart attack, it is likely that the arteries will block off and you will put yourself at risk from a heart attack or developing angina.
- Angina will almost certainly improve if you stop smoking.
- Smoking is the most important cause of furring up of the arteries of the legs. If you do not stop, this could progress so that you find it difficult to walk without stopping and this might necessitate leg surgery.
- Women on the oral contraceptive pill and who smoke are at high risk from developing heart disease and if they cannot stop smoking, they should stop taking the Pill.
- Come to our smoking cessation clinic. Your friends, partner or spouse should help you stop. Cutting down is not stopping.
- You have to set yourself a stop date, understand and be prepared for the effects of withdrawal from a very addictive habit, change your daily routine and get away from the habits associated with smoking. One of these habits may be visiting the pub and so you will have to be prepared to sacrifice parts of your lifestyle that you enjoy. Take one day at a time. It takes several months to 'kick the habit' but it will be worth it.
- Don't worry about putting on weight. You won't if you don't eat differently. When you stop smoking your appetite may increase because you will rediscover your sense of smell and taste. Just be careful, but enjoy!
- There are smoking cessation aids which help but you have to do the main bit.
- Nicotine replacement, bupropion and other new drugs may help if you are having difficulty stopping on your own.
- Nicotine replacements (patches, gum, lozenges, etc.) contain nicotine but are safer than cigarettes.
- Bupropion (Zyban) may help but may not take away completely the urge to smoke. The course lasts for eight weeks and we can give it to you on the NHS. It may give you side effects.

❖ Some people have found hypnotherapy and acupuncture helpful. Do whatever works for you.

Answers to questions about clinical cases

1. There is only a small chance that this patient will be motivated to stop smoking but he should be offered advice and a smoking cessation clinic. The risks of continuing smoking and the benefits of smoking cessation should be discussed with him. All his risk factors should be evaluated carefully and treated. He should be on aspirin if he can tolerate this.
2. Find out if he wants to stop smoking and give him advice and outline the importance to him of stopping. Early after an infarct is a good opportunity to help patients stop smoking using all available techniques. His risk from further cardiac events should be evaluated and if he has not seen a cardiologist, he should be referred.
3. Treat the chest infection, exclude lung cancer and optimise her cardiac treatment. Even though it is unlikely that she will either want or be able to stop smoking, she should be given advice and help in a realistic and sympathetic way.
4. Discuss the vascular and thrombotic risks of the combination of smoking and the oral contraceptive pill and discuss other forms of contraception if she insists on continuing to smoke.
5. She may have coronary artery disease and angina. The history is important but may be difficult to obtain. She should be referred for cardiac evaluation and if the cardiac tests show a low probability of coronary artery disease, she should be investigated for oesophageal reflux and other gastrointestinal problems. It is unlikely that she will respond to advice to stop smoking or undertake a smoking cessation programme, but if you have the resources and she is willing to consider this, she should be offered the opportunity. She may need further specialist input for her other problems.

FURTHER READING

Cochrane Database Syst Rev 2000; (2): CD001008, CD000546, CD000009.

Critchley JA, Capewell S. Mortality risk reduction associated with smoking cessation in patients with coronary heart disease. A systematic review. *JAMA.* 2003; **290:** 86–97.

Ford CL, Zlabek JA. Nicotine replacement therapy and cardiovascular disease. *Mayo Clin Proc.* 2005; **80:** 652–6.

Guidance on the use of nicotine replacement therapy (NRT) and bupropion for smoking cessation. Technology appraisal guidance – No 39. London: National Institute for Clinical Excellence; March 2002.

Handler C, Coghlan G. *Living with Coronary Disease.* London: Springer; 2007. pp. 169–76.

Hirsch AT, Treat-Jacobson D, Landon HA, Hatsukami DK. The role of tobacco cessation, anti-platelet and lipid-lowering therapies in the treatment of peripheral arterial disease. *Vasc Med.* 1997; **2:** 243–52.

Teo KK, Ounpuu S, Hawken S, *et al.* Tobacco use and risk of myocardial infarction in 52 countries in the INTERHEART Study: a case-control study. *Lancet.* 2006; **368:** 647–58.

Tonstad S, Farsang C, Klaene G, *et al.* Bupropion SR for smoking cessation in smokers with cardiovascular disease: a multicentre, randomised study. *Eur Heart J.* 2003; **24:** 946–55.

Yudkin P, Hey K, Roberts S, *et al.* Abstinence from smoking eight years after participation in randomised controlled trial of nicotine patch. *BMJ.* 2003; **327:** 28–9.

Exercise and rehabilitation

NINE

Clinical cases

1. A 57-year-old previously fit man comes to see you one week after an uncomplicated myocardial infarction. He wants to know when he can go back to the gym to do some cycling, treadmill and weightlifting. What advice do you give him?
2. A 38-year-old man joins your practice and tells you that he has familial hypertrophic cardiomyopathy. He would like to join the local gym but he need a doctor's letter confirming that he is fit. What do you do?
3. A 64-year-old man has mild hypertension, a slightly raised cholesterol level and borderline diabetes. He is not at all keen to take any tablets and feels fine. What advice do you give him?
4. A 55-year-old woman who is the carer for her elderly and immobile mother asks you if there is anything that can be done to improve the quality of both their lives. What do you advise?

Benefits of exercise

Regular exercise is inexpensive and has many health and cardiovascular benefits, but most people in the UK do not exercise enough. Physical inactivity is a strong, graded risk factor for coronary heart disease. Physical inactivity doubles the risk of developing cardiovascular disease.

> Physical activity reduces cardiovascular risk and all – cause mortality and has major psychological benefits.
> The benefits of daily exercise are enhanced with moderate alcohol consumption and a low-fat, low-salt diet.

Exercise should be part of the daily activities for people of all ages. Regular exercise underpins primary and secondary prevention. Even a single exercise session has beneficial effects on triglycerides, systolic blood pressure and insulin sensitivity. Walking fast for one hour every day has been shown to reduce cardiovascular events by 28%. As people increase their physical activity, they reduce, in a linear fashion, their cardiovascular risk. The more exercise a person does, the lower their risk of cardiovascular disease.

Primary care health professionals have a pivotal role and responsibility to educate patients and encourage them to exercise.

Regular exercise
✧ prevents atherosclerotic coronary artery disease
✧ reduces mortality after myocardial infarction
✧ improves cardiovascular risk profile
✧ improves exercise capacity in patients with stable angina, heart failure and claudication
✧ lowers blood pressure
✧ prevents development of non-insulin dependent diabetes by lowering blood glucose
✧ helps in treatment of obesity
✧ lowers plasma fibrinogen levels and improves haemostatic parameters
✧ improves lipid profile with increases in HDL cholesterol levels
✧ improves the psychological state, reduces stress and makes people happier.

Effects of regular exercise on cardiovascular risk factors

1. Lipid profile

> Regular exercise reduces lipid levels slightly, and when combined with a low-fat diet, may make drug treatment for hyperlipidaemia unnecessary.

Regular exercise reduces total cholesterol by at least 6%, LDL cholesterol by 10%, and increases HDL cholesterol by 14%. These effects are enhanced by a low-fat diet and weight loss. The beneficial effects of exercise on the lipid profile are most pronounced in overweight patients with high triglyceride levels and low HDL levels. It is difficult to separate the independent effects of exercise because people who are motivated to exercise regularly usually change their diet too.

2. Obesity

Exercise alone has a modest effect on weight loss (approximately 3 kg) over several months. When exercise is combined with diet, most overweight people can lose 8 kg within six months

3. Hypertension

Sedentary people have a 35% greater risk of developing hypertension compared to people who exercise regularly. Regular physical activity delays and may prevent hypertension, and it lowers blood pressure in hypertensives. Gentle cardiovascular exercise (running, cycling) reduces diastolic blood pressure whereas heavy isometric exercise (weight training) may increase systolic blood pressure and left ventricular wall thickness.

> Regular exercise, particularly when combined with weight reduction, may reduce blood pressure sufficiently to make antihypertensive treatment unnecessary in mild hypertensives.

4. Diabetes

Exercise reduces blood glucose and increases sensitivity to insulin. Glucose production by the liver is reduced. Exercise and maintenance of optimal weight prevent the onset of diabetes. Regular exercise reduces glycated haemoglobin by 1%. Antidiabetic medications can often be reduced and sometimes withdrawn in overweight or obese patients who do daily exercise and reduce their carbohydrate intake and lose weight. Daily exercise is as effective as oral hypoglycaemic medication in reducing cardiovascular risk. Exercise is strongly recommended for primary and secondary prevention in diabetics.

5. Smoking

Regular exercise increases the likelihood of successful smoking cessation.

6. Thrombosis

Individuals who are physically active are at lower risk of cardiovascular events. In older people (aged over 60 years), fibrinogen levels are reduced by 13% and active tissue plasminogen activator increased by 140% with regular exercise. These changes have also been seen in younger people and in patients after myocardial infarction. Platelet aggregation is also reduced after regular exercise. Endothelial function is improved and this may also account for the reduced thrombotic tendency after regular exercise.

7. Autonomic effects

Regular exercise increases parasympathetic tone and reduces sympathetic tone and these combined effects may contribute to the reduction in cardiovascular risk. Regular exercise results in a resting bradycardia. Neurally mediated syncope or near syncope in trained individuals is due to a high vagal tone.

8. Psychological effects

People exercise because it makes them feel and look better and fitter. This improves self-esteem, reduces stress and anxiety and is a useful adjunctive therapy for depression. People who exercise regularly are more likely to be concerned about their health and make other lifestyle changes.

9. Haemodynamic effects of exercise

These depend on:
- ⟡ the type of exercise performed – isotonic (e.g. jogging, swimming or cycling), or isometric (e.g. weightlifting)
- ⟡ the muscles used (upper versus lower body)
- ⟡ body position.

Exercise results in increases in heart rate, systolic blood pressure, cardiac output and VO_2 – a measure of energy expenditure and oxygen utilisation. Diastolic blood pressure falls during exercise due to peripheral vasodilatation. These factors lead to an increase in myocardial oxygen demand and this is the basis for exercise stress testing in the evaluation of patients with known or suspected coronary artery disease. The stress test evaluates whether the myocardial blood and oxygen supply can meet the imposed demands.

Normal coronary arteries dilate with exercise but this response is impaired in patients with atheroma. Chest tightness and breathlessness may develop in patients with impaired myocardial oxygen supply and muscle fatigue and breathlessness in those with impaired heart muscle function.

Regular exercise has been shown to improve symptoms and prognosis in patients with heart failure. It is also beneficial in patients with chronic lung disease. Regular exercise, muscle strengthening and spinal flexibility are very useful in people of all ages, particularly in the elderly, and should be recommended to all. Regular exercise makes it easier for elderly people to enjoy a fuller and more active retirement.

Training effects

Regular endurance training results in muscular, cardiovascular and neurohumoral changes which improve functional capacity and strength allowing the individual to exercise more efficiently – to higher workloads with a lower heart rate.

Muscle

There are increases in skeletal muscle mitochondria, myoglobin, capillary density and metabolic enzymes. This promotes aerobic metabolism and increased exercise capacity with lower lactate levels through the use of fatty acids rather than glycogen for energy production. Isometric resistance exercise results in muscle cell hypertrophy.

Cardiovascular

Increases in left ventricular wall thickness result from increases in afterload due to increases in total peripheral resistance and systolic blood pressure. Exercise training results in less myocardial ischaemia in patients with coronary artery disease and this is manifested as an increased exercise time to the onset of angina and an increased exercise time before the onset of ST depression probably because of the mechanisms listed above.

Neurohumoral

The resting heart rate is decreased due to an increase in parasympathetic tone, a decrease in sympathetic tone and a reduction in circulating catecholamines.

Detraining

The benefits of training are lost quickly, within three weeks or less, and this is apparent to all who stop regular exercise for any reason.

Cardiovascular benefits of exercise

There is a progressive decrease in cardiovascular events with increasing intensity of cardiovascular exercise. Walking at 3 mph (5 km/hr) for one hour each day has been shown to reduce the risk of cardiovascular events in healthy women by at least 30% and overall in men and women by as much as 50%. These benefits reflect the favourable effects of exercise on cardiovascular risk factors.

Exercise programmes in primary care
How much?
The benefits of exercise occur when people get breathless and sweaty for 30 minutes every day resulting in an average weekly calorie expenditure of at least 2000 calories. The American Heart Association recommends a weekly calorie expenditure of between 700 and 2000 calories depending on the age and physical ability of the individual. Cycling for 20 minutes against a moderate resistance to 70% of age-predicted maximal heart rate expends approximately 240 calories.

Cycling or walking to work, walking up and down stairs and regular visits to the gym (three times per week) for cycling, rowing, walking or jogging on a treadmill are effective and have major beneficial effects on a person's sense of well-being. Exercise is a very effective 'stress buster'.

People who do moderate exercise (one to two times per week) have a 40% lower cardiovascular mortality risk compared to people who do no exercise. Cardiovascular mortality decreases with increasing daily calorie expenditure and increasing exercise duration. Cardiovascular risk decreases with increasing intensity and duration of exercise. Therefore, the more exercise, the better, in nearly all people. The benefits occur because of the complex interactions of all the proposed mechanisms listed above.

What is moderate exercise?
Walking briskly at 3 to 4 mph for long enough to get breathless is moderate exercise. Slower but sustained walking may be adequate for elderly people because they have a lower peak heart rate and less exercise is required to achieve a training effect. Carrying weights increases the work performed and the exercise intensity. Any exercise is better than none and so walking the dog or playing nine holes of golf is better than sitting, although a round of golf would constitute at most only very low level cardiovascular exercise. Generally, irrespective of the fitness of the individual in question, exercise should be strenuous enough to result in a doubling of the resting heart rate for at least 30 minutes per day.

What exercise to recommend?
It does not matter whether exercise is done inside or outside the home. Treadmills are useful because they allow increases in speed and inclination and result in less impact trauma to the leg and foot joints. Low impact treadmill walking can be achieved by walking up a manageable incline, rather than jogging or running on the level. Cycling and stair climbing should also be encouraged and are useful forms of exercise.

All muscle groups should be exercised and stretched. Isometric exercise should be performed carefully and after guidance and is not recommended for patients with certain cardiac conditions (see below). The level and duration of exercise should be tailored to the individual. This can be done in primary care but requires input from a trainer or physiotherapist or nurse with advice from the GP about the patient's cardiac condition and if there are any restrictions on how much the patient should do. Generally, even in patients with heart failure, coronary heart disease, recent uncomplicated myocardial infarction, or heart surgery, a progressive programme of exercise is safe and beneficial. There are very few absolute contraindications to starting an exercise programme. Unstable angina with rest pain, severe breathlessness at rest or critical aortic stenosis, preclude exercise training.

Exercise should be part of the treatment for all stable cardiac conditions. Where there is concern or doubt about its safety, patients can have an exercise test under supervision in primary care, or referred to hospital for assessment. Exercise testing early after myocardial infarction identifies patients at low risk from subsequent cardiac events. It provides the information for an exercise prescription and reassures the patient and their family about their condition, which should encourage them to exercise daily.

Both walking and vigorous exercise are associated with substantial reductions in the incidence of cardiovascular events in post-menopausal women irrespective of race, ethnic group, age, or body mass index.

> Daily exercise is as important as a daily aspirin for patients with coronary heart disease, and as important for patients with heart failure as a daily diuretic.
>
> Exercise should be combined with a reduced calorie intake (to 1500 Kcal per day), a fat intake reduced to 30% of total energy uptake, avoidance of trans-fats, increased fibre intake to 30 g per day, and avoidance of sugars and excess salt.

Exercise for the elderly and physically less able

Although it may be impossible for elderly, bed-bound or chair-bound people to perform conventional cardiovascular exercise, they may nevertheless be able, with instruction and encouragement, to have passive exercise and breathing exercises. Elderly people can remain active and independent for longer if they are encouraged to remain physically and mentally active.

Home-based or healthcentre-based programmes can be arranged with enthusiastic helpers and some guidance from experienced professionals. These may be physiotherapists or nurses who have experience from a neurological or cardiac rehabilitation unit.

In whom is exercise potentially dangerous?

Sudden cardiac death due to ventricular tachycardia and ventricular fibrillation may occur in young, fit athletes with inherited or congenital cardiovascular abnormalities. It may also occur in patients with coronary artery disease or structural heart disease, for example, severe hypertrophic cardiomyopathy or aortic valve stenosis.

1. Sudden cardiac death in young athletes

The risk is low, probably less than 1 in 200 000. Death typically occurs either during or immediately after exercise.

It is not standard practice in the UK to screen all athletes for cardiovascular disease because of the high prevalence of false-positive results and the cost implications. High-risk individuals should be evaluated on the basis of the nature and severity of the cardio-vascular condition and the classification of the sport involved.

The current recommendations for participation in competitive sports are summarised in Table 9.1.

TABLE 9.1 Recommendations for participation in competitive sports

DIAGNOSIS	RECOMMENDATIONS
Hypertrophic cardiomyopathy	Should not participate in competitive sports
Congenital coronary artery anomalies	Should not participate in competitive sport unless they have been revascularised and have no residual ischaemia
Wolff-Parkinson-White syndrome	Can participate if no structural heart disease, palpitation or tachycardia
	Can participate after successful accessory pathway ablation
Dilated cardiomyopathy	Cannot participate in competitive sports
Coronary heart disease	Can participate in the absence of symptoms, ischaemia, induced arrhythmia, normal left ventricular function
Marfan's syndrome	Only low-level sports allowed if there is aortic root dilatation. Can participate in the absence of family history of sudden death and aortic root dilatation
Myocarditis	No competitive sport until cardiac function is normal
Aortic stenosis	Mild stenosis (<20 mmHg) – can participate
	Moderate stenosis (<40 mmHg) – low-intensity sport only
	Severe stenosis (>40 mmHg) – cannot participate in any competitive sport

2. Screening young athletes at high risk

Those at high risk include those with symptoms, the abnormalities listed in Table 9.1, and those with a family history of premature cardiac disease or sudden death. Screening should include history and examination, resting ECG and 2D echocardiogram to look for structural and functional abnormalities. Stress testing is required to evaluate those with suspected coronary artery disease. Ambulatory ECG recordings are required for those with palpitation.

Seeding an exercise philosophy for life in the young

British people are exercising more than their parents and grandparents and this encouraging trend should continue if schoolchildren are encouraged look upon exercise as a 'life skill'. This would necessitate political will and support. Competitive school sports should be seen as part of a step towards this long-term lifestyle. Engagement in the fun and enjoyment of sport, comradeship and teamwork should be encouraged rather than deprecated. Sport is naturally competitive and should no longer be considered as elitist. It is beneficial for all, irrespective of a person's ability. Children should be encouraged to participate in the sport that they most enjoy. Getting children and young people into the 'exercise habit' is a key part of helping them develop physically and emotionally and learn skills which they should use throughout their life.

Cardiac rehabilitation

Approximately 300 000 people suffer a heart attack each year in Britain, and myocardial infarction claims 140 000 deaths per year. Cardiac rehabilitation involves patient education, comprehensive secondary prevention, psychological measures to reassure patients and exercise training. It has proven benefits after myocardial infarction, resulting in a 34% reduction in cardiac mortality and a 29% reduction in recurrent infarction. Ideally, cardiac rehabilitation after infarction should start at the time of hospital admission. It also has benefits in patients after coronary artery surgery and in heart failure. It is most useful in patients who have lost confidence after a heart attack or find their cardiac condition difficult to accept or understand.

Cardiac rehabilitation can be performed safely, effectively and cheaply in primary care. The quality of the programme depends on the enthusiasm and skills of the multidisciplinary staff and, the effectiveness of cardiac rehabilitation depends on the attitude of the patients and their families.

What is involved?

The patient

The patient should be willing, motivated and interested in cardiovascular prevention and the measures needed to improve their prognosis. They should be prepared to use the six- to eight-week programme, with two attendances per week, as a springboard for continuing self-help healthcare and a lifelong commitment to regular exercise. Patients must take long-term, full-time control of their lives and be committed to all components of a healthy lifestyle.

The staff

The sessions are usually run by a nurse and/or a physiotherapist. Medical input adds an extra dimension. This team may be complemented by interested, trained and educated lay helpers who can provide useful reassurance particularly if they have recovered from a heart attack or coronary artery surgery themselves and have been through a rehabilitation programme. The staff should receive training in a good unit, have appropriate life-support skills and knowledge of defibrillation, be given updated literature and teaching aids, and encouraged to share the expertise and experience of staff working in other units.

Patients at high risk may need a hospital-based programme and access to staff with advanced life-support training. The general thrust of each component of the programme can be modified depending on the type of patients attending. Each member of the team should be encouraged to inject their own personality and, when appropriate, humour and warmth into the sessions. Without this, the sessions can be lifeless and 'sterile' and have little impact and consequently little long-term effect.

Pre-enrolment evaluation

The patient's history can be obtained by proformas and practice records. The blood pressure and resting heart rate should be recorded. Signs of heart failure should be sought. Patients with angina at rest, important arrhythmias, uncontrolled hypertension, or pulmonary oedema at rest should be assessed by a doctor and treated before they start the rehabilitation programme. Exercise is contraindicated in patients with critical aortic stenosis and exertional symptoms.

Facilities

A suitable space, resuscitation facilities, exercise cycles and/or treadmills or other exercise equipment including stairs, rowing machines or elliptical training machines can be used for cardiovascular exercise. Gentle weights or medicine balls are useful for some patients. There should be complete and regularly checked resuscitation equipment and the necessary drugs.

The programme

Patients should be taught the principles and practice of cardiovascular prevention and be allowed to ask questions about their health, medical history, life stresses and anxieties. They may need specialist help for depression or psychological problems including personal, marital or sexual problems.

The programme offers the opportunity for the primary care team to review the patient's medical history, risk-factor status, diet and medication and drug compliance.

The long-term benefits of a rehabilitation programme depend on the ability of the patient to accept and follow the advice given but this is difficult for most people and the short-term benefits often disappear within a year. New information from clinical trials will result in new recommendations and this information should be passed on to patients.

Primary care is probably the most effective arena where primary and secondary prevention can be offered and updated on a continuing basis but this has major resource implications. Effective long-term risk reduction requires lifelong commitment from patients and primary care input.

Risk of death during cardiac rehabilitation

This is approximately 1 per 170 000 patient hours of participation and this may be lower or no different than the risk among patients not involved in a cardiac rehabilitation programme.

Exercise training for patients with coronary heart disease

Until the advent and widespread use of aspirin, β-blockers, angiotensin-converting enzyme inhibitors, thrombolytics and acute coronary angioplasty, regular exercise and other risk-factor interventions were the only effective secondary preventative therapies after myocardial infarction. Exercise training for two to six months following myocardial infarction combined with smoking cessation and dietary changes, reduced total mortality by 20%, cardiovascular mortality by 22%, fatal reinfarctions by 25%, and sudden death at one year by 37%. Current drug treatments have greatly reduced mortality and morbidity after infarction and so the benefits of exercise training may not be as great but are still worthwhile when combined with other interventions.

In patients with mild to moderate angina, exercise training improves exercise capacity by the haemodynamic mechanisms mentioned above.

Exercise for patients with congestive heart failure

Exercise training improves exercise capacity but not survival.

Exercise for patients with peripheral vascular disease

Regular exercise increases claudication distance by 180% or approximately 225 m to the onset of pain and should be strongly recommended to all suitable patients with claudication. The greatest improvement is seen when patients are exercised to maximal levels – maximum tolerated pain. The mechanism for this is unclear but may relate to opening of collaterals. These results are as good as surgical and pharmacological therapies. Patients can exercise by walking or perhaps more conveniently during all seasons, on a static exercise cycle or treadmill.

The Athlete's heart and cardiovascular responses

Patients may ask about the potential cardiac dangers of regular training and sport. This would include élite athletes and those who participate in high-level competitive sports. It is important for primary care physicians to be aware of the effects of exercise on the heart, which clinical and investigative findings are abnormal and require further evaluation, and those which are normal and do not.

It is important to distinguish Athlete's heart from hypertrophic cardiomyopathy. A diagnosis of hypertrophic cardiomyopathy excludes an athlete from competition with adverse financial, psychological and physical consequences. Patients with hypertrophic cardiomyopathy typically have severe left ventricular hypertrophy on echocardiography but some have only slight hypertrophy making it difficult to distinguish the two conditions, which may also co-exist.

ECG changes

Approximately one-third of élite athletes have an abnormal ECG and most of them have no underlying cardiac disease and are at low risk.

The enhanced parasympathetic and reduced sympathetic tone resulting from training may cause:

✧ resting bradycardia
✧ increased sinus arrhythmia (increased heart rate variability with breathing)
✧ prolonged PR interval (first-degree heart block)
✧ steep take off of the ST segment

✧ voltage criteria of left ventricular hypertrophy is particularly likely in slim endurance athletes, e.g. long-distance runners

✧ atrioventricular conduction delay

✧ Mobitz type I second-degree atrioventricular block which may be apparent on the ECG.

Notes:

✧ Mobitz type II second-degree atrioventricular block is rare in athletes and is more likely to be due to conduction tissue disease.

✧ Wolff-Parkinson-White syndrome is more common in endurance athletes and the risk of sudden death in symptom-free individuals is low.

The most common ECG changes seen in athletes are ST-segment abnormalities (increased voltages, early take-off) and widespread T-wave changes. These may pose a diagnostic and management problem and require a specialist opinion because they may also signify other cardiac disease. When combined with echocardiographic evidence of symmetric left ventricular hypertrophy, these ECG changes of Athlete's heart must be distinguished from the steep T-wave inversion and classic asymmetric hypertrophy of hypertrophic obstructive cardiomyopathy (HOCM) which may co-exist in approximately 1% of athletes and is the most common cause of sudden death in young people. The situation is complicated when HOCM results in symmetric left ventricular hypertrophy (as may be seen in hypertension). Therefore, it is important to detail the patient's athletic activities, blood pressure and ECG findings if an echocardiogram is requested. Where there is diagnostic doubt, the patient should be referred.

Vasovagal syndrome

Compared with strength-trained athletes, endurance-trained athletes have an increased tendency to faint due to postural hypotension. The mechanisms include enhanced vagal tone, reduced sympathetic tone and increased lower-limb venous capacity. Tilt table responses may be abnormal. Individuals who experience troublesome symptoms should be referred for a specialist opinion and may require dual chamber pacing to protect them from fainting due to an impaired heart rate response in the presence of a low blood pressure.

Left ventricular hypertrophy

Significant left ventricular hypertrophy (more than 12 mm; upper limit of normal = 11 mm) is rare. It occurs in 2% of athletes, principally in rowers, canoeists, cyclists, distance runners who perform regular isometric and isotonic large-muscle bulk exercise. It is an adaptation to exercise and reversible after a few months. Severe wall thickening (greater than 16 mm) is unusual in athletes and is more probably due to hypertrophic cardiomyopathy. Causes other than endurance exercise should be considered in athletes with more than mild left ventricular hypertrophy. Approximately 15% of individuals may develop increased left ventricular cavity size suggestive of dilated cardiomyopathy.

Cardiac murmurs

Athletes may have a larger stroke volume and increased blood velocity due to vigorous cardiac function. The commonly heard systolic murmur in young slim people may be normal and due to increased flow across both the right and left ventricular outflow tract or, in athletes, due to vigorous cardiac function. Systolic murmurs are usually benign. Diastolic murmurs are always pathological. Echocardiography is helpful in investigating the possibility of structural heart and valve disease.

TABLE 9.2 Comparison of Athlete's heart and hypertrophic cardiomyopathy (HCM)

	ATHLETE'S HEART	HCM
Echocardiography		
Maximal left ventricular wall thickness	mild <13 mm	≥ 16 mm
LV hypertrophy type	concentric	Asymmetric but variable
LV cavity size	large	small
Diastolic function	normal	impaired
Left atrial size	normal	dilated
Regression of hypertrophy with detraining	regression	no regression
Family history	nil of hypertrophy	more likely
ECG	*see* above	septal Q-waves, deep T-wave inversion, left axis

Risk and causes of sudden cardiac death in athletes

This is extremely rare – averaging annually at approximately 1 per 500 000 young people. It is more common in males. This is lower than the prevalence of hypertrophic cardiomyopathy in young people (0.2%).

The most common causes of death of young individuals who have died suddenly during exercise are hypertrophic cardiomyopathy (over 50% of cases) and coronary artery anomalies (13%) and less commonly congenital aortic stenosis (6%) and myocarditis (7%).

Atherosclerotic plaque rupture, acute myocardial infarction and ventricular fibrillation are the most frequent cause of sudden death in adult athletes. The annual risk of death in symptom-free healthy joggers had been estimated at 1 in 18 000 but this may be similar to or less than the risk of death in a similar age-matched symptom-free non-jogging population.

The risk of death is increased in previously sedentary individuals with unrecognised cardiovascular risk factors who take up vigorous exercise. The risk is very low in individuals who have exercised regularly over a long period and who have no risk factors.

Identifying high-risk individuals before they start exercise training

Exercise testing before starting exercise training is recommended to detect reversible ischaemia in individuals with a history of coronary artery disease (angina, infarction revascularisation). It is not necessary in low-risk, symptom-free individuals because of the low prevalence of obstructive coronary artery disease.

A significant proportion of athletes who suffered exercise-related cardiac events had prodromal symptoms which were ignored. Therefore, a full cardiac evaluation including stress testing is recommended for athletes who develop cardiac symptoms, those with a family history of an inherited cardiac disorder or a family history of 'unexplained' premature death below the age of 40 years (*see* Table 9.1). Therefore, athletes with palpitation, syncope, chest pain or surprising shortness of breath require specialist referral and full evaluation.

Advice for patients

◇ Regular exercise is good for you. It halves the risk of developing heart disease and stroke and should be part of a healthy lifestyle including modification of all cardio-vascular risk factors.

◇ The more exercise, the better. Get hot, sweaty and breathless for 30 minutes per day. Any form of exercise that is convenient, comfortable and can be performed regularly is appropriate. Get into the habit and make it a fixed part of your daily routine.

◇ Elderly people should walk, swim or cycle to comfortable levels every day. It keeps them fitter, more alert and independent for longer. Any exercise is better than nothing.

◇ Exercise and attaining the optimum weight reduces the risk of diabetes, and make you feel better, more energetic and less depressed.

◇ Exercise reduces the risk of developing high blood pressure and is important part of its treatment.

◇ Exercise is part of the treatment for heart failure and for patients recovering after heart attacks but should be done carefully after an exercise test.

◇ Exercise lowers the risk of developing osteoporosis.

◇ Stretching and improving the strength in your arms and legs will make it easier for you to remain active when you get older.

Answers to questions about clinical cases

1. If he is symptom free and has no signs of heart failure on examination, arrange a symptom-limited exercise test if he has not already had one. If he has a satisfactory exercise time with no ischaemia and a normal blood pressure he is at low risk for subsequent cardiac events and could go back to the gym, but should take it easy. He should avoid heavy weightlifting for four weeks. Check his medication, fasting lipids (if not already done) and ask him if he would like to join a rehabilitation course. If he develops symptoms or ischaemia, he should be referred back to the cardiologist for further investigation and coronary angiography.

2. Confirm with his previous GP or specialist that the diagnosis is correct. Patients with hypertrophic obstructive cardiomyopathy are advised not to participate in competitive sports. He should be advised that moderate exercise is safe and he should

be instructed by an experienced sports trainer that he can jog or cycle gently but not over-exert himself by exceeding 70% of his age-predicted maximal heart rate. He can swim, walk, and play golf and tennis. It is difficult to restrict young active men. We need to educate patients that sudden vigorous exertion resulting in rapid increases in heart rate and systolic blood pressure are potentially dangerous but this depends on the nature and severity of the underlying heart disease.

3. It is possible that regular daily exercise combined with a careful diet might delay the time he requires tablets. The only way to find out is to try. He may need some guidance on an exercise prescription and will require monitoring.

4. This is a difficult and common problem and may require a multidisciplinary approach. It may be possible to make her mother more mobile and independent and to improve the fitness and morale of the daughter if they both did some exercise. The mother will need careful evaluation of her musculoskeletal (arthritis) and neurological systems (Parkinson's disease, cerebrovascular disease), a general medical evaluation (haematological, biochemical and thyroid status) and home assessment. Passive exercise and activities to increase her muscle tone and power are important. Standing, sitting and general mobility exercises should be given under the supervision of a physiotherapist experienced working with people of this age.

FURTHER READING

26th Bethesda Conference. Recommendations for determining eligibility for competition in athletes with cardiovascular abnormalities. January 6–7, 1994. *J Am Coll Cardiol.* 1994; **24:** 845–99.

Atterhog JH, Jonsson B, Samuelson R. Exercise testing: a prospective study of complication rates. *Am Heart J.* 1979; **98:** 572–79.

Billman GE, Schwartz PJ, Stone HL. The effects of daily exercise on susceptibility to sudden cardiac death. *Circulation.* 1984; **69:** 1182–9.

Coats AJ. Exercise training in heart failure. *Curr Control Trials Cardiovascular Med.* 2000; **1:** 155–160.

Handler C, Coghlan G. *Living with Coronary Disease.* London: Springer; 2007.

Huston TP, Puffer JC, Rodney WM. The athletic heart syndrome. *N Engl J Med.* 1985; **313:** 24–32.

Manson JE, Greenland P, LaCroix AZ, *et al.* Walking compared with vigorous exercise for the prevention of cardiovascular events in women. *N Engl J Med.* 2002; **347:** 716–25.

Maron BJ. Athlete's Heart and Sudden Cardiac Death. In: Topol EJ. *Comprehensive Cardiovascular Medicine.* Philadelphia: Lippincott-Raven; 1998.

Maron BJ. Hypertrophic cardiomyopathy: a systematic review. *JAMA.* 2002; **287:** 1308–20.

Mittleman MA, Maclure M, Tofler GH, Sherwood JB, Goldberg RJ, Muller JE. Triggering of acute myocardial infarction by heavy physical exercise. Protection against triggering by regular exertion. Determinants of Myocardial Infarction Onset Study Investigators. *N Engl J Med.* 1993; **329:** 1677–83.

Noakes TD. Heart disease in marathon runners: a review. *Med Sci Sports Exerc.* 1987; **19:** 187–94.

O'Connor GT, Buring JE, Yusuf S, Goldhaber SZ, Olmstead EM, Paffenbarger Jr RS, Hennekens

CH. An overview of randomised trials of rehabilitation with exercise after myocardial infarction. *Circulation.* 1989; **80:** 234–44.

Pedersen JØ, Heitmann BL, Schnohr P, Grønbaek M. The combined weekly influence of leisure-time physical activity and weekly alcohol intake on fatal ischaemic heart disease and all-cause mortality. *Eur Heart J.* 2008; **29:** 204–212.

Powell KE, Thompson PD, Caspersen CJ, Kendrick JS. Physical activity and the incidence of coronary heart disease. *Ann Rev Public Health.* 1987; **8:** 253–87.

Siscovick DS, Weiss NS, Fletcher RH, Lasky T. The incidence of primary cardiac arrest during vigorous exercise. *N Engl J Med.* 1984; **311:** 875–7.

Thompson PD, editor. *Exercise and Sports Cardiology.* New York, NY: McGraw-Hill; 2001.

Thompson PD, Moyna NM. The therapeutic role of exercise in contemporary cardiology. *Cadiovasc Rev Rep.* 2001; **22:** 279–84.

Vongvanich P, Paul-Labrador MJ, Merz CN. Safety of medically supervised exercise in cardiac rehabilitation center. *Am J Cardiol.* 1996; **77:** 1383–5.

Diabetes and the heart

TEN

Clinical cases

1. A 76-year-old overweight diabetic woman with a long history of hypertension comes to see you complaining of aching legs and cold feet. What do you do?
2. A 38-year-old Asian man with type 1 diabetes complains of chest pain which does not sound like angina. He is worried about his heart because his father died from a heart attack aged 65 years. What do you do?
3. An 88-year-old man with hypertension and diabetes presents with angina. What do you do?
4. A 64-year-old man, who has had coronary angioplasty and leads a full and busy life, is overweight, and you diagnose hypertension and diabetes. What advice do you give him?
5. A 60-year-old hypertensive (treated with bendrofluazide and lisinopril), obese woman has inadequately controlled diabetes with early-morning glucose levels of >8 mmol/l and a high HbA$_1$c of 8.5%. What do you do?

Definition of diabetes

Diabetes is a metabolic disorder characterised by chronic hyperglycaemia with disturbances of carbohydrate, fat and protein metabolism resulting from defects of insulin secretion, insulin action, or a combination of both. Diabetes, whether type 1 or type 2, is associated with the development of organ damage due to microvascular disease and increases the risk for cardiovascular, cerebrovascular and peripheral artery disease.

> Most diabetics die from cardiovascular disease.

Type 1 diabetes

Type 1 diabetes is due to a lack of endogenous insulin secretion from the pancreas. It usually presents in childhood but can present at any age. Patients with type 1 diabetes are prone to ketoacidosis and weight loss. It is associated with other autoimmune diseases. It presents as either acute or subacute ketoacidosis. Patients feel unwell, weak, hyperventilate, have weight loss, thirst, and pass a lot of urine.

Type 2 diabetes

The cause of type 2 diabetes is more complex. It is usually detected during screening in primary care and less commonly in hospital. Type 2 diabetes is more common in people aged over 40 years but it is becoming more prevalent in young people. Type 2 diabetes results from a combination of genetic predisposition, unhealthy diet, physical inactivity, and increasing weight. It is therefore largely preventable.

> Daily exercise and significant weight loss can prevent, or at least delay, the onset of type 2 diabetes. Simple lifestyle interventions are inexpensive and effective.

Diagnostic criteria of diabetes

The normal fasting plasma glucose is <6.1 mmol/l with a two-hour post-glucose-load plasma glucose of <7.8 mmol/l.

Diabetes can be diagnosed in a symptomatic patient if a fasting glucose is >7.0 mmol/l or the glucose concentration two hours after a glucose load (oral glucose tolerance test) is >11.1 mmol/l. Do not diagnose diabetes if only one fasting blood sample is >7.0 mmol/l. At least two consistent results should be obtained.

Impaired glucose tolerance is a fasting plasma glucose of <7.0 mmol/l or a two-hour post-glucose-load plasma glucose of >7.8 mmol/l.

Oral glucose tolerance test

Early stages of hyperglycaemia and asymptomatic type 2 diabetes are most accurately diagnosed by an oral glucose tolerance test which provides a fasting and a two-hour post-glucose value.

If in doubt about the diagnosis, do an oral glucose tolerance test. Ask the patient to fast overnight. They should come to the health centre in the morning for a fasting glucose blood test. They then drink 75 g of glucose dissolved in 300 ml of water. Two hours later, the venous plasma glucose is measured. A level of >11.1 mmol/l is diagnostic.

An intermediate state of impaired glucose tolerance (IGT) or subclinical glucose intolerance is a fasting glucose of >6.1 mmol/l and <7.0 mmol/l.

> Patients with impaired glucose tolerance are at greater cardiovascular risk than normoglycaemic patients.

Gestational diabetes

The diagnostic criteria are the same for other types of diabetes. Women with gestational diabetes are at increased risk from diabetes later.

Glycated haemoglobin (HbA$_1$c)

HbA$_1$c is used to measure glycaemic control and the efficacy of treatment, and the patient's compliance with diet and medication. It represents the average blood glucose during the preceding six to eight weeks (the life of a red cell). HbA$_1$c is not recommended as a diagnostic test for diabetes. A normal HbA$_1$c value does not exclude diabetes or impaired glucose tolerance.

Increasing prevalence of type 2 diabetes

Diabetes is becoming increasingly common in the UK due to the British (and almost worldwide) lifestyle of taking too little exercise, eating an unhealthy high-calorie diet, drinking excess alcohol, resulting in obesity. It is estimated that 195 million people throughout the world have diabetes and this will increase to 330 million or possibly as many as 500 million by 2030. Fifty per cent of diabetics are undiagnosed.

Of the two million people in the UK who have diabetes, 85% have type 2 diabetes. Most of these are adults, but there is an increasing incidence of diabetes in children. Children who do little exercise and who eat a lot of carbohydrate and sugar are a high-risk group and require special attention. The prevalence of type 2 diabetes is higher in people of Afro-Caribbean descent and South Asians living in the UK and Europe.

Screening for diabetes

It is important to identify diabetes in symptom-free patients, particularly those with coronary heart disease. All adults and perhaps overweight children, and those with a family history should be routinely screened for diabetes. This can be done cost effectively by asking patients to complete a questionnaire focusing on weight, family history, diet, and other risk factors, and using previous blood tests and other clinical data (for example, for women who may have had hyperglycaemia during pregnancy), to help identify people at risk of developing diabetes later. Blood testing is the most accurate.

Patients with coronary heart disease but without known diabetes should be screened with an oral glucose tolerance test.

Diabetes and cardiovascular risk

Macrovascular disease, resulting in coronary heart disease, is the major cause of death in diabetics. More than 75% of diabetics aged over 40 years will die from a cardiovascular cause and are more likely than non-diabetics to die from their first cardiovascular event.

The Framingham Study showed that, after controlling for the effects of major cardiovascular risk factors, diabetes increased the relative risk of developing coronary heart disease to 66% in men and to 20% in women followed up for 20 years. Female diabetics appear to be more vulnerable to cardiovascular risk than males. The risk of cardiovascular disease and mortality from myocardial infarction is increased further in diabetics with microalbuminuria and proteinuria or any other risk factor.

> Diabetes as a risk factor for cardiovascular events is the equivalent of coronary heart disease.
>
> Diabetics who have coronary heart disease are at particularly high risk from cardiovascular death. Women are at even greater risk than men.
>
> Diabetics, whether they have coronary heart disease or not, should be considered for the same preventative interventions as patients with coronary heart disease.
>
> Diabetics constitute a particularly high-risk group who require early diagnosis, energetic and effective cardiovascular risk-factor identification and lower thresholds for intervention.
>
> Diabetics are two to three times more likely to die from cardiovascular disease than non-diabetics. Diabetes appears to be a more potent risk factor in women.
>
> Diabetes is the strongest single-risk factor for stroke, increasing the risk in men by four times and in women five times. The outcome of stroke is worse in diabetics.
>
> All adults should be screened for type 2 diabetes.
>
> Impaired glucose intolerance is a risk factor for cardiovascular disease.

The mortality of adult diabetics without coronary heart disease is similar to that of non-diabetics with coronary heart disease, suggesting that type 2 diabetes confers a risk similar to that of established coronary heart disease. After a first coronary event, 50% of patients with diabetes may die within one year, and half of those die before they reach hospital. One-third of young, insulin-dependent (type 1) diabetics die from coronary heart disease by the age of 50 years. Subclinical glucose intolerance also increases cardiovascular risk and so all patients with one or more cardiovascular risk factors should be screened for diabetes and monitored.

Compared with non-diabetics, diabetics are at greater risk from:
✧ obstructive coronary artery disease
✧ peripheral vascular disease
✧ renal artery stenosis
✧ retinopathy
✧ neuropathy and autonomic dysfunction
✧ angina
✧ myocardial infarction and its complications, including death
✧ heart failure
✧ cerebrovascular disease.

Diabetics are more likely to require:
✧ coronary artery surgery
✧ coronary angioplasty

✧ peripheral vascular intervention

✧ long-term medical treatment and monitoring of risk factors.

Diabetics have a poorer short- and long-term success rate following:

✧ coronary angioplasty (although this may be improved with new adjunctive medications and stents)

✧ coronary artery surgery which has been the preferred approach to revascularisation for certain subsets of patients

✧ myocardial infarction.

Pathology

Vascular problems

Diabetes increases atherogenesis by several mechanisms including glycosylation of proteins and lipoproteins and oxidative damage, prothrombosis, impaired fibrinolysis and high levels of atherogenic LDL particles. Compared with non-diabetics, diabetic patients are more susceptible to accelerated atherogenesis and obstructive and unstable vascular disease with a greater tendency to plaque rupture, platelet activation and thrombosis. These processes underlie the clinical consequences listed below.

Renal problems

These increase cardiovascular risk and mortality and the incidence of hypertension, which compounds the risks. Renal problems are determined mainly by genetic influences and only partially by glycaemic control.

Diabetes results in a pre-nephropathy phase characterised by subclinical albuminuria (microalbuminuria detected by radio-immunoassay and not dipstix) and subsequently nephropathy with proteinuria, decreasing glomerular filtration rate and increasing blood pressure. Cardiovascular mortality is 37 times greater in patients with nephropathy and nearly all of them have significant coronary artery disease; it is four times greater in patients without proteinuria. This is the rationale for angiotensin-converting enzyme inhibitors in diabetics.

Microalbuminuria is associated with a prothrombotic profile with a raised LDL, decreased HDL, raised lipoprotein (a) and raised activity of plasminogen activator inhibitor, factor VII and plasma fibrinogen.

Global risk assessment and management

Obesity, diabetes, hyperlipidaemia and hypertension often co-exist. A vigorous, global approach to risk-factor improvement in diabetics reduces cardiovascular risk and improves prognosis. Estimation of absolute cardiovascular risk using the Joint British Societies' risk chart or Cardiac Risk assessor computer programme is helpful in rationalising treatment decisions.

Multifactorial-risk-factor assessment and intervention combined with long-term monitoring for the recognition and management of diabetic complications, therefore, constitute a major, ongoing burden of work in primary care.

Recent trials in diabetics have confirmed the benefits of vigorous lipid lowering, and tight blood pressure and blood sugar control in reducing cardiovascular morbidity, retinopathy and proteinuria. Diabetic patients will often be taking more than one form of medication because they are likely to derive considerable benefit from treatment of all their risk factors.

> The benefits of risk-factor intervention are commensurately greater in diabetics and this is the rationale for lower thresholds for risk-factor interventions in diabetics.

Waist circumference vs body mass index (BMI)

Waist circumference is used as the clinical screening factor for metabolic syndrome because it is a more powerful predictor of metabolic risk than BMI. It is also easier to use because patients generally know their waist measurement but not their BMI.

The metabolic syndrome

The well-recognised association of a raised blood sugar, dyslipidaemias, and hypertension in obese people has been recognised for several years. It is probably due to insulin resistance. The International Diabetes Federation definition is central obesity (waist girth >94 cm for men and >80 cm in women) plus any two of the following four factors:

◆ raised serum triglycerides >1.7 mmol/l or specific treatment for this
◆ fasting blood glucose 5.6 mmol/l or >100 mg/dL or previously diagnosed diabetes. If fasting glucose >5.6 mmol/l, an oral glucose tolerance test is recommended
◆ hypertension with systolic >130 mmHg or diastolic >85 mmHg, or treated hypertension
◆ reduced HDL cholesterol <1.0 mmol/l or any specific treatment for this abnormality.

This relatively recently characterised syndrome is common, affecting around 25% of men and women and is due to insulin resistance. The prevalence increases from 7% in people aged 20 to 30 years to 40% in people aged 60 years and older.

It appears that obese patients have insulin resistance which then tends to progress with resulting dyslipidaemias, hypertension and/or type 2 diabetes. Metabolic syndrome and its complications may be missed in individuals with low or borderline levels of the diagnostic biochemical characteristics but it is advisable to keep them under surveillance. Coronary heart disease in young patients may be explained by the metabolic syndrome rather than a genetic abnormality. A large proportion of patients with metabolic syndrome progress to diabetes and conversely, a large proportion of patients diagnosed as 'diabetic' several years ago, would now at presentation be diagnosed as having metabolic syndrome.

The metabolic syndrome is associated with vascular inflammation with raised C-reactive protein levels suggesting that it may not be simply due to glucose intolerance and insulin resistance.

The aim of treatment of the metabolic syndrome is the same as treating diabetes, namely to prevent morbidity and mortality due to cardiovascular disease. Relatively modest lifestyle changes can substantially reduce the risk for type 2 diabetes in mildly hyperglycaemic people. The management of patients with vascular disease and the metabolic syndrome centres on vigorous risk-factor correction.

> Lifestyle changes, particularly a low-carbohydrate and low-fat diet, weight loss and daily exercise, are recommended for patients with the metabolic syndrome. It is important that patients understand that vascular disease may be present at the time diabetes is diagnosed.

Statins and a fibrate may be needed to raise the HDL, and lower the triglycerides and LDL cholesterol. Metformin and thiazolinediones are insulin sensitisers and may play a role in patients without diabetes but at present there is little data to support this approach.

Educating and supporting patients to manage their diabetes

Patient education and motivation are the most important aspects of the long-term management of patients with diabetes and those at risk of developing diabetes. It requires intensive, regular counselling about diet, weight, exercise, and monitoring and tight control of diabetes and its complications. Patients have to be fully engaged and in control of a lifelong lifestyle modification, and monitoring and controlling their diabetes. These processes should be audited in the practice.

In primary care, specialised clinics should aim to provide continuing, long-term education and training for patients and their families to explain their condition, and help them manage their diabetes and all other risk factors. Patients are more likely to take control of their condition, and compliance with medication and lifestyle interventions will be improved if they understand what diabetes is, how it can affect them and how a disciplined lifestyle can improve their chances of a longer and healthier life. This may be achieved with patient self-help groups guided by interested primary care clinicians who may have a special interest in diabetes.

Principles of diabetes management

These have changed over the last few years following the publication of major trials, including the United Kingdom Prospective Diabetes Study Group (UKPDS) and the Heart Outcomes Prevention Evaluation (HOPE) Study Investigators. Our understanding of the pathophysiology and natural history of diabetes and its complications has resulted in increasingly aggressive risk-factor intervention and this is likely to continue.

Epidemiological extrapolation of data from the UKPDS study showed that a 1% reduction in HbA$_1$c would be associated with a 21% decrease in the risk of any diabetic complication, a 21% decrease in death due to diabetes, a 31% decrease in microvascular complications and a 14% reduction in the risk of macrovascular events.

> Strict glycaemic control reduces microvascular and macrovascular complications and cardiovascular complications.
> Lifestyle measures are at least as effective as glucose-lowering drugs.

Diabetics are a high-risk group and those with one or more additional risk factors, very high risk. Management of diabetes requires the identification of diabetics and vigorous and effective management of the following:

- Those with established vascular disease (previous myocardial infarction, myocardial revascularisation, cerebrovascular and/or peripheral vascular disease).
- Those, particularly females, who have one or more cardiovascular major risk factors, particularly hypertension, hyperlipidaemia, obesity.
- Diabetics with microalbuminuria.
- Diabetics with nephropathy (macroalbuminuria).
- Diabetics with retinopathy.
- Asians.
- Patients with poor glycaemic control.

Management should focus on reducing absolute risk using lower thresholds for intervention and the following targets:

- The early identification of glucose intolerance in patients at risk of cardiovascular disease (family history or one or more cardiovascular risk factors).
- Sympathetic, clear, tailored and reinforced dietary advice.
- Target HbA_1c <6.5%.
- Fasting glucose target level <6.0 mmol/l. The post-prandial peak glucose target for type 1 diabetics is 7.5–9.0 mmol/l, and for type 2 diabetics it is <7.5 mmol/l.
- Achievement of optimal weight (BMI <25), and a waist measurement for men of <94 cm and for women of <80 cm.
- Metformin as first-line treatment in overweight type 2 diabetics.
- Tight blood pressure control at or below 130/80 mmHg (this is often not possible).
- Smoking cessation.
- Encouraging regular daily exercise of 30 minutes or more.
- Aggressive lipid lowering.
- ACE inhibition with or without an angiotensin II antagonist for hypertension, heart failure, post-myocardial infarction, vascular disease, microalbuminuria or multiple risk factors.
- Aspirin treatment for those both with cardiovascular disease and those without.
- Annual screening for microalbuminuria and retinopathy are mandatory.
- Insulin is the gold standard therapy for type 1 diabetes, aiming at an HbA_1c <6.5%.

Smoking

Diabetics are likely to derive greater benefit from smoking cessation than non-diabetics. Therefore, smoking cessation is particularly important in diabetics reducing the risk of myocardial infarction by 50% within one year of quitting.

Exercise and prevention of cardiovascular disease in diabetics

Regular physical activity reduces the risk of cardiovascular disease and death from any cause in diabetics. Diabetics should be encouraged to walk or cycle to work or as part of their day. Moderate exercise reduces cardiovascular mortality by 17% and a high level of daily exercise reduces cardiovascular mortality by 40%.

> In patients with type 2 diabetes, daily exercise is as effective as drug treatment in reducing blood glucose levels and reducing cardiovascular risk. Daily exercise is recommended for primary and secondary prevention in diabetics who should be encouraged exercise every day.

Hypertension

Diabetic patients should be checked and monitored carefully for hypertension. Hypertension affects 40% of patients with type 2 diabetes by the age of 50 years and 60% of patients aged 75 years or older. The UKPDS trial showed that tight blood pressure control reduced diabetes-related death and microvascular events and stroke and heart failure, but not myocardial infarction.

> All patients, whether diabetic or not, should be treated if the blood pressure is >160/100 mmHg.
>   Target blood pressure is <130/80 mmHg unless the patient has microalbuminuria or macroalbuminuria, when the target is lowered to <125/75 mmHg.

Choice of drug for diabetic patients with hypertension

Most diabetics will need more than one antihypertensive drug to achieve target blood pressure levels. The aim of treatment is to achieve target blood pressure levels without adverse effects.

UKPDS showed that atenolol and captopril were similarly effective in reducing the incidence of diabetic complications. However, angiotensin-converting enzyme inhibitors and angiotensin II receptor blockers have advantages over other drugs and are the drugs of first choice in patients with microalbuminuria and also in the following situations:

✧ For patients with heart failure. Diuretics may also be necessary.

✧ Patients should be switched to an angiotensin II receptor blocker if they cannot tolerate an angiotensin-converting enzyme inhibitor which is usually because of a ACE-inhibitor associated cough.

✧ Blood pressure control may be improved by the addition of an angiotensin II receptor blocker to an angiotensin-converting enzyme inhibitor although there will be no further improvement in microalbuminuria.

✧ Afro-Caribbean patients respond poorly to β-blockers and angiotensin II receptor blockers and usually respond better to the calcium channel blockers and diuretics.

✧ β-blockers, combined when necessary with calcium antagonists, are useful in patients with angina, post-myocardial infarction or in patients who cannot tolerate other drugs.

Hyperlipidaemia

Type 2 diabetes typically results in a raised triglyceride level and a reduced HDL cholesterol level.

Prevention targets for cholesterol and lipid fractions for diabetics are the same as for secondary prevention targets in patients without diabetes:

✧ total cholesterol <3.5 mmol/l
✧ fasting triglyceride <2.0 mmol/l
✧ LDL cholesterol <1.8 mmol/l
✧ HDL cholesterol >1.1 mmol/l
✧ total cholesterol : HDL cholesterol <3.0.

> The vascular event rates in adult diabetics of all ages, both males and females with and without vascular disease, are reduced with high-dose statins which should therefore be considered in all diabetics. Fibrates should be used in addition for hypertriglyceridaemia.

Most diabetics will require a statin to achieve these targets, and possibly a fibrate and ezetimibe.

Statins are as effective in reducing cardiovascular events in diabetics as they are in non-diabetics, but because the absolute risk of cardiovascular events is higher in diabetics, the number needed to treat is lower.

Secondary prevention strategies are the same for diabetics as non-diabetics, but treatment thresholds are lower.

Renal function

Renal function should be evaluated before undertaking procedures using radiographic contrast media, which can precipitate renal failure in patients with renal impairment. Pre-procedure or pre-operative fasting may also induce renal failure in susceptible patients.

The use of non-cardiac drugs with potential renal side effects (for example, non-steroidal anti-inflammatory drugs), should be used very cautiously and renal function should be monitored

Diabetic control

The UKPDS trial showed that tight glycaemic control (glycosylated haemoglobin of <7%) reduced microvascular complications. Insulin and dextrose infusions may need to be given to patients who are not allowed to eat perioperatively.

Four main steps have been proposed in treating type 2 diabetes.

1. Lifestyle changes

✧ Assess and optimise the patient's lifestyle and psychological state.
✧ If target HbA_1c is not achieved, go to step 2.

2. Monotherapy

Metformin

Metformin is the only available biguanide. It decreases gluconeogenesis and increases utilisation of glucose and there has to be some insulin secretion for it to work. It is the drug of first choice in overweight patients (the majority of type 2 diabetics). It may cause renal impairment and so should be omitted on the day of surgery, or of procedures using contrast material. It does not usually cause weight gain, but can cause gastrointestinal side effects.

Introduce metformin in patients with BMI >25 kg/m^2 unless:
✧ there are contraindications or metformin is poorly tolerated
✧ there is renal impairment (creatinine >130 μmol/l)
✧ there is a risk of renal impairment because of history of cardiac or hepatic failure.

Sulphonylureas

If any of these contraindications apply, and in patients with BMI <25 kg/m^2, introduce an insulin secretagogue (e.g. sulphonylurea). Sulphonylureas augment insulin secretion. They are used in patients who are not overweight and in those who cannot tolerate metformin. They may cause hypoglycaemia, abnormal liver function tests, cholestatic jaundice and hepatitis, and unwanted weight gain. They are contraindicated in ketoacidosis, and severe hepatic or renal disease. Use as low a dose as possible.

If HbA_1c target is not achieved, go to step 3.

3. Combination therapy

Consider metformin + insulin secretagogue (standard sulphonylurea or prandial glucose regulator) combination therapy if:
✧ there are no renal problems or tolerability issues.

Consider metformin + glitazone if:

✧ metformin + insulin secretagogue is contraindicated or not tolerated
✧ patient has BMI >25 kg/m².

Thiazolidinediones

Thiazolidinediones (rosiglitazone, pioglitazone) reduce peripheral insulin resistance. They are used alone or with metformin or a sulphonylurea in patients who cannot tolerate a combination of metformin and sulphonylurea, or in whom either metformin or a sulphonylurea is contraindicated. They are also used as add-on therapy for patients with high glycated haemoglobin levels despite maximum doses of metformin plus a sulphonylurea. Some endogenous insulin secretion is essential. Thiazolidinediones have similar efficacy as insulin in decreasing glycated haemoglobin by two percentage points, but are more expensive. Weight gain (3–4 kg) and gastrointestinal side effects may occur, but HDL cholesterol levels increase by 10%. Thiazolidinediones are contraindicated in inflammatory bowel disease and severe hepatic and renal disease, and there is an increased risk of oedema, congestive heart failure, and fractures in women. There is uncertainty about the safety of rosiglitazone in patients with coronary heart disease. Pioglitazone is preferred to rosiglitazone for patients with coronary heart disease and those who have more than one cardiovascular risk factor.

Consider insulin secretagogue + glitazone if:

✧ there is renal impairment (serum creatinine >130 μmol/l)
✧ there is a risk of sudden deterioration in renal function because of a history of cardiac or hepatic failure
✧ either metoprolol or gliclazide is not tolerated or is ineffective.

If HbA$_1$c target is not achieved, go to step 4.

4. Insulin therapy

Reassess psychological issues and any lifestyle change, and give or obtain appropriate support.

Discuss and agree treatment change to insulin.

Initiate 10 IU basal insulin (NPH insulin at bedtime; insulin glargine at any time, but at the same time of day each day).

✧ Titrate dose to achieve target fasting blood glucose (4.0–7.0 mmol/l) slowly over a period of weeks.
✧ Continue treatment with metformin.
✧ Discontinue other antidiabetic agents.
✧ Review other medications/interventions as appropriate.

If HbA$_1$c target not achieved, introduce short or rapid-acting insulins prior to meals and review other medications.

Exenatide

This is a new glucagon-like peptide (GLP-1) receptor agonist. It lowers glucose levels by stimulating insulin secretion and inhibiting glucagon secretion. It enhances gastric emptying and satiety leading to weight loss. It is comparable in efficacy to other antidiabetic treatments. It can be added to metformin and a sulphonylurea in patients with type 2 diabetes who continue to have suboptimal control. Side effects include nausea and rarely, pancreatitis. It is expensive and long-term data are not available.

Angina and coronary artery disease

Diabetes results in accelerated atherosclerosis. Diabetes is considered to be as potent a risk factor as cardiovascular disease. This is because diabetics without coronary heart disease are likely to have a similar rate of myocardial infarction and cardiovascular death and other events as non-diabetics who have had an infarct. Diabetics have a blunted or diminished appreciation of angina but, compared with non-diabetics, are more likely to have coronary heart disease. Silent ischaemia and infarction are therefore more common in diabetics.

Compared with normoglycaemia, hyperglycaemia is associated with a worse outcome in patients with acute coronary syndromes. Tight control of diabetes reduces long-term mortality in patients with acute coronary syndromes. This is done with insulin and monitored with HbA_1c.

Medical treatment

The principles of medical treatment of acute coronary syndromes and angina in diabetics are similar to those governing treatment in non-diabetics, but co-existing risk factors should be treated aggressively and at lower thresholds, in accordance with absolute risk estimation.

- Smoking cessation, weight loss, dietary control and exercise are crucial.
- Prophylactic short-acting and long-acting nitrates, calcium antagonists, β-blockers and, in resistant cases, potassium channel openers are used.
- Aspirin (75–150 mg a day) is recommended to all diabetics with vascular disease and also to those without vascular disease although this is not based on randomised trial evidence. Clopidogrel 75 mg may be used in addition in some patients.
- Angiotensin-converting enzyme inhibitors improve endothelial function in patients with coronary artery disease. The HOPE study showed that ramipril produced significant reductions in the risk of the combined outcome of death, myocardial infarction and stroke and nephropathy. Angiotensin-converting enzyme inhibitors should be prescribed for diabetic patients with vascular disease, more than one risk factor, or microalbuminuria.
- Statins are recommended for secondary prevention and reduce major cardiovascular events and the need for myocardial revascularisation by 40%. This is mainly due to reductions in LDL cholesterol. For secondary prevention, the LDL target for diabetics and other high-risk patients is <1.8 mmol/l.

Myocardial revascularisation

Revascularisation strategies in diabetics with angina are more complicated because the underlying coronary artery disease is more likely to be diffuse, affecting the whole length of the artery. This makes angioplasty and coronary artery surgery technically difficult and an unattractive option because of the higher short-term and long-term risks. Infection risks are higher. Tight glycaemic control during the perioperative and long-term post-operative phases are important and influence outcome.

Coronary artery bypass surgery

Diabetes is an independent predictor of short-term morbidity and long-term survival after coronary artery surgery. This probably relates to the higher risk of widespread and progressive vascular disease and associated renal disease. Technical problems including manipulation of an atheromatous and calcified aorta resulting in emboli, and graft insertion into a diffusely diseased and narrowed distal coronary artery contribute to perioperative and long-term morbidity and mortality from infection, graft occlusion and myocardial infarction.

Renal failure may develop in patients with pre-existing diabetic renal disease. It may also occur when coronary artery surgery is performed shortly after the use of large volumes of contrast medium for angiography or angioplasty.

Infection and slow healing of the leg vein harvest sites may present difficult problems for the primary care team.

Coronary angioplasty

Before the advent and wider use of coated coronary artery stents and glycoprotein IIb/IIIa inhibitors in diabetics, coronary artery bypass surgery was shown to offer diabetic patients a better five-year survival mainly because of the high restenosis rates after angioplasty in diabetics.

Associated renal disease and renal artery stenosis pose an increased risk of renal failure with the use of radiographic contrast media during angiography.

Diabetics are more likely to have diffuse multivessel coronary artery disease rather than having focal lesions.

Peripheral vascular disease increases the technical difficulties of vascular access and post-procedure complications. Patients with carotid and cerebrovascular disease are at risk from cerebrovascular events. Patients should be screened for associated vascular disease before revascularisation is performed so the risks of the chosen approach are minimised. Emboli from the aorta to the brain and legs are more likely in diabetics.

Combined angioplasty and coronary angioplasty

Hybrid approaches using both angioplasty and minimally invasive direct coronary artery bypass grafting using internal mammary arterial conduits are a relatively new approach which may offer improved short- and long-term outcomes although there are no data to support this at present.

Myocardial infarction

The risk of myocardial infarction in increased to 50% in men and to 150% in women, and 30% of diabetics die from infarction.

Silent ischaemia and autonomic neuropathy may explain the absence or blunting of angina, or atypical symptoms of angina and myocardial infarction, in diabetics. The complications of infarction, including sudden death, are more common in diabetics because of the nature of their coronary artery disease, their atherogenic and prothrombotic predisposition and late or non-presentation to emergency medical care for resuscitation, thrombolysis and intervention. Patients who survive the acute ischaemic event are more likely to have larger infarcts and associated heart failure and cardiogenic shock.

Tight blood sugar control using insulin has been shown to improve survival after infarction but the UKPDS trial showed only a borderline reduction in the risk of infarction. Other current secondary preventative treatments in the management of acute myocardial infarction apply to and should be used in diabetics: primary coronary angioplasty; medical thrombolysis, and other medical interventions including aspirin, β-blockers and statins. Angiotensin-converting enzyme inhibitors should be used to prevent left ventricular remodelling and heart failure and microvascular complications.

Diabetic cardiomyopathy

Occasionally, diabetics may develop heart failure due to a diabetic cardiomyopathy and this is distinct from the much more common situation of muscle damage resulting from myocardial infarction.

Screening diabetic patients for coronary heart disease

At present, this is recommended for patients only prior to major non-cardiac surgery and renal transplantation where the presence of important coronary artery disease and ischaemia may adversely affect the operative success and where myocardial revascularisation would improve the outcome.

The most accurate and direct approach to assessing coronary anatomy is to perform coronary angiography rather than non-invasive imaging. Stress testing may be helpful in certain patients but nuclear perfusion imaging has a low sensitivity (5–10%) in asymptomatic patients.

Advice for patients

✧ Your diabetes puts you at greater risk from furring up of all your arteries and so we must work together to make sure that your diabetes is very tightly controlled. You will have a lower risk of heart trouble, stroke or circulation problems in your legs if your diabetes is well controlled. This involves a lot of work and self-discipline but it is worth it. It is important that you understand how you can control your future with lifestyle modification.

✧ All the factors which contribute to arterial furring up need continuous vigorous attention. This includes smoking, blood pressure, cholesterol, and perhaps most importantly, your weight and your diet.

✧ Please speak to one of our team about how to achieve a safe weight and how else you can lower your blood sugar simply and effectively without tablets.

✧ There are several tablets which will help you and we need to make sure that they are suitable for you. If your blood sugar remains too high despite tablets, you may need insulin.

Answers to questions about clinical cases

1. She needs to be assessed for vascular disease affecting her legs and also for coronary heart disease and carotid artery disease. She should have her glucose state checked, together with her blood count, lipid status and renal function. She should be referred to the peripheral vascular team. If she has not seen the diabetologists recently, she should be reviewed. An ECG might show signs of ischaemia or hypertension. She will need help and advice about her diet, glucose control and exercise. Her blood pressure will have to be tightly controlled. She should be on an angiotensin-converting enzyme inhibitor if possible, plus aspirin and other appropriate medication.

2. Examine his heart and blood pressure, feel his peripheral pulses, check his glucose and lipid status and arrange an exercise test. If he has a good exercise performance and no signs of reversible ischaemia, then he can be reassured. Estimate his absolute coronary risk and initiate prevention treatment as necessary.

3. He needs a comprehensive assessment and hopefully his symptoms will be adequately controlled on medical treatment. Angioplasty is an option to be considered if this is not possible.

4. His hypertension and newly diagnosed diabetes may respond to weight loss and he needs to understand this. If it doesn't, then he will need medication. Take a full dietary history and details of how much and how often he exercises. Give him clear, detailed advice about a low-fat, low-carbohydrate diet. If he is able and willing, he should also be given an exercise prescription. He should be seen frequently, initially perhaps once a week for weighing, and to check his blood pressure and blood sugar. In most cases, significant weight loss combined with regular – preferably daily – exercise, should be effective and he could avoid taking long-term medication.

5. Good tight diabetic control with a glycated haemoglobin of <6.5% and attention to all risk factors is crucial in order to reduce cardiovascular complications. She should be asked about her diet, her attitude to weight loss and exercise, all cardiovascular risk factors. Examine her heart, lungs, blood pressure, urine, ECG, waist circumference, fundi, and signs of a peripheral neuropathy. A detailed dietary history should be taken. A carefully supervised low-carbohydrate diet and regular daily exercise are important. Check for microalbuminuria, dyslipidaemia. She should have a statin if her LDL is >1.8 mmol/l or her total cholesterol is >4.5 mmol/l. Her blood pressure should be <130/80 mmHg or lower if she has renal impairment. She is already taking metformin and gliclazide. Aspirin is recommended if she has vascular disease. There are three options: add pioglitazone; add neutral protamine insulin before bedtime;

add exanatide twice daily. There are pros and cons involved with each approach and these can be discussed with a diabetologist.

FURTHER READING

Reviews

Barnett AH. Treatment intensification in patients with type 2 diabetes. *Diabetes Obes Metab.* 2008; **Suppl 1:** iii.

McGuire DK, Granger CB. Diabetes and ischaemic heart disease. *Am Heart J.* 1999; **138:** S336–S375.

The Task Force on Diabetes and Cardiovascular Diseases of the European Society of Cardiology (ESC) and of the European Association for the Study of Diabetes (EASD). Guidelines on diabetes, pre-diabetes, and cardiovascular diseases: executive summary. *Eur Heart J.* 2007; **28:** 88–136. *(Note: This paper contains 711 references.)*

Timmis AD. Diabetic heart disease: clinical considerations. *Heart.* 2001; **85:** 463–9.

Epidemiology

Fuller JH, Shipley MJ, Rose G, *et al.* Mortality from coronary heart disease and stroke in relation to degree of glycaemia: the Whitehall study. *BMJ.* 1983; **287:** 867–70.

Kannel WB, McGee DL. Diabetes and cardiovascular risk factors: the Framingham study. *Circulation.* 1979; **59:** 8–13.

Stamler J, Vaccaro O, Neaton, *et al.* Diabetes, other risk factors, and 12-yr cardiovascular mortality for men screened in the multiple risk factor intervention trial. *Diabetes Care.* 1993; **16:** 434–4.

Myocardial revascularisation

Marso SP, Lincoff AM, Ellis SG, *et al.* Optimizing the percutaneous interventional outcomes for patients with diabetes mellitus: results of the EPISTENT (Evaluation of Platelet IIb/IIIa Inhibitor for Stenting Trial) diabetic substudy. *Circulation.* 1999; **100:** 2477–84.

The Bypass Angioplasty Revascularisation Investigation (BARI) Investigators. *N Engl J Med.* 1996; **335:** 217–25.

Risk-factor intervention

National Cholesterol Education Program (NCEP) Third Adult Treatment Panel (ATP-III). *JAMA.* 2001; **285:** 2486–97.

United Kingdom Prospective Diabetes Study (UKPDS) Group. Efficacy of atenolol and captopril in reducing risk of macrovascular and microvascular complications in type 2 diabetes (UKPDS 39). *BMJ.* 1998; **317:** 713–20.

United Kingdom Prospective Diabetes Study (UKPDS) Group. Intensive blood-glucose control with sulphonylureas or insulin compared with conventional treatment and risk of complications in patients with type 2 diabetes (UKPDS 33). *Lancet.* 1998; **352:** 837–53.

United Kingdom Prospective Diabetes Study (UKPDS) Group. Tight blood pressure control and risk of macrovascular and microvascular complications in type 2 diabetes (UKPDS 38). *BMJ.* 1998; **317:** 703–13.

Yusuf S, Sleight P, Pogue J, *et al.* (for The Heart Outcomes Prevention Evaluation (HOPE) Study). Effects of ramipril on cardiovascular and microvascular outcomes in people with diabetes mellitus: results of HOPE study and MICRO-HOPE substudy. *Lancet.* 2000; **355:** 253–9.

Treating type 2 diabetes

Goldberg RB, Holman R, Drucker DJ. Management of Type 2 Diabetes. *N Engl J Med.* 2008; **358:** 293–7.

Patient advice

Handler C, Coghlan G. *Living with Coronary Disease.* London: Springer; 2007. pp. 151–7.

Index